Running
WITH THE WHOLE BODY

Running
WITH THE
WHOLE
BODY

A 30-Day Program to Running Faster with Less Effort

By
JACK HEGGIE

Photography by
Donna M. Hornberger

Somatic Resources
Berkeley, California

North Atlantic Books
Berkeley, California

Everyone—particularly those over the age of 35 or who have known heart or blood pressure problems—should have a complete physical examination by his or her physician before beginning a strenuous exercise program such as running.

Running With the Whole Body: A 30-Day Program to Running Faster with Less Effort

Published by
North Atlantic Books   Somatic Resources
P.O. Box 12327   and   P.O. Box 2067
Berkeley, California 94712   Berkeley, California 94702

Cover photograph by Richard Blair
Cover design and production by Catherine E. Campaigne

Running With the Whole Body: A 30-Day Program to Running Faster with Less Effort is sponsored by the Society for the Study of Native Arts and Sciences, a nonprofit educational corporation whose goals are to develop an educational and crosscultural perspective linking various scientific, social, and artistic fields; to nurture a holistic view of arts, sciences, humanities, and healing; and to publish and distribute literature on the relationship of mind, body, and nature.

Library of Congress Cataloging-in-Publication Data
Heggie, Jack.
    Running with the whole body : a 30-day program for running faster with less effort / Jack Heggie.
        p.   cm.
    Originally published: Emmaus, Pa. : Rodale Press, © 1986
    Includes bibliographical references (p.   ).
    ISBN 1-55643-226-7
    1. Running—Training.   2. Feldenkrais method.   I. Title.
GV1061.5.H44   1996
796.4'26—dc20   96-24591
                                                         CIP

1 2 3 4 5 6 7 8 9 / 00 99 98 97 96

Acknowledgments

I'd like to offer a special thanks to the students in my running classes at Brookhaven College in Dallas, upon whose
learning experiences many parts of this book are based.
Their interest, support, and willingness to put up with my
often unconventional ideas and exercises gave life to this
project. I hope they got as much out of my classes as I
did working with them.

Contents

Preface

This book grew out of my studies with Dr. Moshe Feldenkrais, the Israeli scientist who devised a system of psy-
chophysical movement known as the Feldenkrais Method.
The approach used here draws upon ideas that he developed over many decades of teaching.

    The floor exercises are taken from his system of im-
proving human functioning, which he called Awareness
Through Movement. The actual arrangement of the exercises, the standing exercises, and the idea that the shoulders and arms are the "drive point" for proper motion of
the legs and feet are all of my own devising.

Introduction
To the 1996 Edition

When *Running With The Whole Body* was first published in 1986, few people had ever heard of the Feldenkrais Method of Awareness Through Movement, and only a handful of Feldenkrais practitioners had completed the four year training required to practice the Method in the United States.

A decade later almost a thousand Feldenkrais practitioners use the method in the USA; more than double that figure practice worldwide. Many people have found that the Method gives relief from pain, enhances mobility, and improves posture and breathing. Athletes commonly use it to improve performance, and its use by physical therapists for injuries has grown by leaps and bounds. Feldenkrais' ideas about improving ability by increasing awareness instead of just trying harder are gaining greater acceptance.

I have received many letters since 1986 from runners young and old. They tell their stories of how applying the Feldenkrais Method to running helps them run faster, reduce and sometimes eliminate pain, and breathe more deeply and evenly. The letters talk about rediscovering a simple renewed zest for running.

Use of the functional connection between the arms and shoulders, and the hips and legs, which I call the Drive Point, is crucial for many other activities besides running. For example, in order to use the newly popular in-line skates, a good understanding of the Drive Point is essential. If you skate, try activating the Drive Point while wearing your skates, but keep your elbows fairly straight. The same goes for ice skating — keep your elbows straight as you experiment with this upper-lower body connection.

The Drive Point is also essential for skiing, both downhill and cross country. If you are a cross country skier, try the exercises in Chapters 10 and 11 while wearing your skis on snow. In *Skiing with the Whole Body* I describe how to use the Drive Point in downhill skiing.

And finally, there's walking. Walking is one of the easiest and simplest exercises for the human body. It's especially good for older adults. Nature has designed our bodies so that they will be self- regulating if we use them correctly. *Running with the Whole Body* is a refresher course in how nature intended us to run and walk. Cats know the proper way of running for cats. Dogs and horses know the proper way of running for them, just as every human body knows the proper way of running and walking for humans. But many life conditions, ranging from poor habits, stress, injuries and impairments, a poor self-image and lack of focus can obscure this "forgotten" knowledge. These awareness exercises will help you to find again your own natural way of walking and running.

If you are more of a walker than a runner, or want to change your exercise program to include more walking, you can still use the exercises in the book. At any place in the text where "running" is mentioned, just substitute the word "walking."

You will soon find that your walking has become smoother, easier, more rhythmical, and less tiring — more like you would like it to be.

Happy running — and walking, skating, skiing.

— Jack Heggie
Boulder, Colorado
September, 1996

Introduction

I was born to run. I just wasn't born to run very well.

Oh, I tried. For years I worked grimly at running. Every day I huffed and strained through workouts. Every night I massaged my unhappy muscles. I leapt at "miracle" training programs the way wistful dieters leap at grapefruit pills.

But I didn't improve my times. And I never enjoyed myself. What I *did* do was watch runner after runner cruise serenely past me. As their shorts faded into the distance, I cursed, my feet slapped awkwardly against the pavement, and my sore body begged to be taken home.

Then, one day, it happened. I was running laps in Albuquerque, New Mexico. Far behind me, blue mountains shimmered in the sunlight, like hills in a dream. Dry heat washed over my skin, and as I ran, I forgot to think about whether I was using "proper" form. I forgot to think about anything except the beauty of the day. My arms pumped and my hips swiveled. And suddenly, I was running. Really running. It was effortless. It was fun. I was fast!

But it wasn't fun and I wasn't fast for long. The next day, in fact, when I went out and tried to recreate that flowing stride, I couldn't. The harder I tried, the sloppier my running became.

That incredible day had been the best thing that had ever happened to my running. Frustrated and angry, I pulled off my running shoes, hurled them toward the track's infield, and plopped down in the grass to sulk. Why was I running so poorly today when I'd run so easily yesterday?

As I lay there, I could see myself as I'd run yesterday. I

knew that I usually looked ungainly. My arms flailed while my legs were stiff. But I could feel now, all through my body, how liberating yesterday's run had been. I could see myself whizzing around the track, shoulders and hips working in harmony with my legs. I'd looked like a real runner for the first time in my life.

I sat bolt upright in the grass. That was it. Yesterday, for the first time, I had run *with my whole body*. I realized that I'd been approaching my training all wrong for years. One day I'd concentrated on leg placement or stride length, another day I'd worried about pumping my arms right. But what I'd pretended was that those limbs work independently of one another. They don't. It's not the individual motion of a runner's feet, legs, hips, arms, or shoulders that's important to running, but the *connections between them*. Only by running with our whole bodies can we ever approach our potential as runners.

The Feldenkrais Connection

This insight struck me as I lay in the infield that day. Actually, it should have hit me long ago. Since 1980 I'd been studying the theories of Moshe Feldenkrais, the Israeli scientist who believed that by working with movement you can improve the organization of your entire nervous system.

My own background in physics had first drawn me to Feldenkrais and convinced me of the validity of his work. But only now did I see how the Feldenkrais Method could be applied to running. Obviously, running is a whole-body undertaking. Hips and shoulders should be as involved as legs. But most of us deliberately sabotage our running by ignoring the incredible strength of the hips, shoulders, and spine. Worse, we ignore the fact that physiologically, neurologically—even psychologically—the different parts of our bodies are inalienably interconnected. They affect one another. Knee pain is as likely to be a symptom of poor arm movement as it is of foot problems.

Until we free our bodies of the bad habits we unconsciously impose on them and begin cultivating an "understanding" between all their parts, we can never run as fast or as far as we might.

Injury-Free Running

I began to put all of this to use in my own running. And I began to run better. My mileage doubled, then tripled. But unlike most runners who rapidly increase their mileage, I never injured myself. Why? I'm sure it's because I'd had a second, perhaps even greater insight that day on the track in Albuquerque. While discovering that the Feldenkrais Method could be adapted to running, I'd also realized that it couldn't simply be slapped onto my running. You don't improve at any physical task by analyzing or hollering at your body. You improve by listening to it.

I'd never known this because I'd never listened to my body before. Like most people, I'd thought running could be analyzed, attacked, and thus improved. I'd thought it could be logically handled. It can't.

Most of the movement of the body is not controlled by your conscious mind at all. Have you ever tripped and, before you thought about reacting, righted yourself and continued unconcernedly along? You were, for that one moment, using what I call your "moving mind." Your moving mind guides you when you're running well. But it can't be forced into improving your running. It must be taught—properly.

My point is that you can't consciously think yourself into becoming a better runner. If you're reading this book, you probably have already read a series of coaching manuals. They might have advised you to strike the ground first with your heel, roll around to the outside of your foot, and then up onto your toes for maximum propulsion. If so, they were right. This is the way most good runners' feet strike the ground.

But if you go out now and consciously practice running this way, you won't be successful for long. If you concentrate on your feet, you'll ignore your shoulders. If you think about your shoulders, you'll start to hold your breath. Or a dog will bark at you and you'll forget everything except how to flail away and get home as fast and as awkwardly as you can.

Instead, you should think less. The exercises in this book will teach your "moving mind" to recognize whether your hips, shoulders, back, or arms are misaligned and which connections between them are being misused. When you go out on the road to put this knowledge to use, you should think only about movement and rhythm in general, about how easily your body can be in sync with itself.

The beauty of my approach to running is that it's personalized. You don't impose someone else's theories about "proper" form onto yourself. Instead, you work with your own body to discover *your* best running form. This may be the same form that Bill Rodgers has. Or it may not be. If you carefully watch world-class runners race, you'll notice that they all have tics and eccentricities in their style. Their running isn't homogenized. Each allows his body, with all its individual talents and defects, to decide how best to propel him across the finish line.

Thirty Days to Better Running

You can do the same. For four years I've been teaching running classes using the Feldenkrais Method. My students have ranged from talented competitors to novices so inexperienced in running that they showed up in tennis shoes. But after a few sessions, all these people were beginning to run better. And because I think anyone can do the same—even without a teacher—I've set forth the curriculum of my running classes in this book.

By practicing the exercises here, you'll be a better runner in just 30 days. All you need is a carpeted living room or bedroom floor—anywhere that you can stretch out—and a willingness to open yourself to the sensations of your own body. After the first chapter, I think you'll be a quicker, smoother runner. And after a month, when you've learned what it really means to run with your whole body, you'll begin to leave panting, straining runners in your wake. You'll know what it feels like to fly.

How to Use This Book

In the following chapters you will find a simple yet very powerful and effective method of improving the way you run. Each chapter consists of a lesson that will improve some aspect of the overall organization of your body. Here are some important points to keep in mind as you practice these lessons:

1. When doing the exercises, make slow, light, easy motions. *Never* strain. If you sweat and strain to do the movements, you'll just be practicing sweating and straining, and you 'll get pretty good at it. This will defeat the purpose of the exercises—which is to reduce strain and effort and to increase efficiency.

2. You can wear whatever you like to do these exercises, as long as it is comfortable and does not restrict your movement. Loose pants, warmups, shorts and a T-shirt, unitard, or leotard and tights all work well.

3. When you make a specific movement, such as lifting the head or moving one hip, make a very small, slow motion. Move only as far as is easy and then return to the initial position. After a few repetitions, you'll find that the range of the easy part of the motion increases considerably by itself, without you having to figure out consciously how to improve the motion.

4. Repeat each motion about 25 times. This allows the part of the mind responsible for movement to absorb the motion and to learn to do it efficiently. If a movement seems difficult or produces any pain, however, you may do fewer than 25 repetitions. Do some of the other lessons in the book and then come back to the movement that was difficult; you'll probably find that it's now easier and doesn't cause any pain.

5. As you move, pay attention to your breathing. If you find that you are holding your breath, it probably means you are straining without knowing it. Reduce the size of the motion you are making and let yourself breathe easily.

6. Don't try to do all the lessons at once. Do one and then wait a day or two for what you have learned to sink into your body. Then do the next lesson, wait another day or two, and so on. In between lessons, pay attention to how you move as you go about your daily activities. You'll probably be surprised to find subtle yet profound improvements in all of your movements.

7. Each exercise is thoroughly illustrated with photographs. It is best, however, to use the photographs only as a general guide. Refer to the directions in the text for specific instruction on how to do the motions and use the photographs only if you have a question about the directions. Although each exercise is to be done on both the right and left sides of the body, only one side is illustrated.

8. Allow yourself plenty of time to do an exercise, about an hour to an hour and a half. This allows the nervous system plenty of time to absorb the new information it is learning.

9. After you have completed the book, you can go back to the first lesson and go through all the lessons again. On the second time through you'll discover even further improvements in the quality of your movements. The more you learn, the more you are able to learn.

1

Feet, Hips, and Shoulders

If you do it well, running can be one of the best exercises for your body. Watch an expert runner and you'll see what I mean. His movements are fluid and graceful, and his stride, while long and powerful, comes with ease. His whole body is at work while he runs, which is why running is so beneficial for him.

You don't have to be an expert runner to move gracefully and easily. But many runners move *so* poorly that all they get from running are aches and pains. Why is this? To answer this question, let's take a look at that incredible machine that enables us to run: the human body.

Unique in the animal kingdom, the human body stands upright. This has its advantages and disadvantages, for while it frees our hands for manipulation and carrying, it also imposes strict balance requirements on us. In fact, it takes a human infant much longer than any other animal to learn to walk and run, and part of the reason is because the human baby has to learn to deal with its two-legged, upright stance.

What does this mean to the aspiring runner? Because of these balance requirements, the human body has developed an elegant means of staying upright while walking and running. Unfortunately, not many runners use the upright stance and balancing mechanisms to full advantage. As a result, they do not run as fast, as far, or as smoothly as they might.

Look at a human body in motion. The right foot and leg advances to take a step, putting all of the weight on the left foot. This results in a curious thing: When the right foot pushes forward, the weight of the right leg moving forward pushes back against the body and causes it to turn to the right.

If you stand up and have a friend push backward against your right hip, you'll be able to feel this clearly. The push will move you back, of course, but it will also cause you to turn to the right a little.

When running or walking, however, we don't actually turn to the side every time we take a step. In fact, when a good runner moves his right foot forward, his right hip actually moves forward also, not backward. Why is this?

A physicist would say that to prevent this turning motion, the twisting push exerted on the body by the advancing leg, which he would call torque, must be balanced by an equal push in the opposite direction. In the human body, this opposite push is provided by the motion of the shoulders and arms. And it is this hip-shoulder connection that many runners do not use as well as they might.

When attempting to sprint, for example, we almost always direct most of our effort into the legs and ignore the arms and shoulders; this pushes the body off balance with each step. When this happens, the part of the nervous system that is responsible for balance will try to bring us back to an upright position and we wind up fighting ourselves—and using much more effort than we need to.

In addition, most runners who ignore their arms and shoulders when they run also stiffen their chest muscles. This inhibits breathing and cuts down on maximum possible running distance. Finally, such misuse of the body puts undue stress on the knees, ankles, and feet, and may lead to aches and pains—and possibly more serious problems in these areas.

Fortunately, the problem is easy to correct if you approach it in the right way. In many cases, what may appear to be multiple problems with your running—aching knees, shallow breathing, and a slow, awkward gait—might actually be only one problem. You might be able to correct the problem in a few hours just by learning to use your body in a more efficient, synergistic way as you run—that is, by learning to run with your *whole* body.

Begin by exploring the motion of your body while you walk, to see what you can learn. Find a place where you can walk for a few hundred feet on flat ground in a straight line. Start walking, and as you walk, pay attention to your right foot and hip. Try to discover how your right hip moves as your right foot moves forward to take a step. (Photo 1-1)

You'll probably have to spend a few minutes working at this before you get a good feeling for just how the right hip moves as the right foot moves forward. Although the motion is simple, most of us are not used to paying attention to ourselves in this way while moving. Much of the time we have our attention on the purpose of the movement, not on the movement itself.

Keep walking until you can easily feel the motion of the hip. As the right foot moves forward, does the right hip move forward or backward with respect to the rest of your body?

After walking for a while, you should be able to notice that as the right foot moves forward to take a step, the right hip also moves forward a bit—that is, the hip follows the foot. If you pay careful attention, you may discover that your walk changes a little as you begin to identify the motion of the hip.

You may also feel that your hip moves up toward your head and a little bit inward toward the center of your body as it goes forward. The hip actually does move a little in these directions, although the exact motion is different for

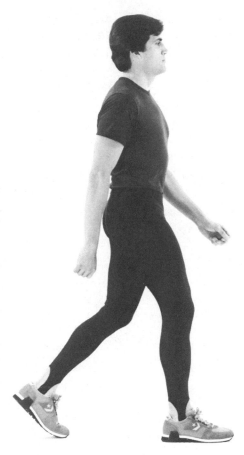

Photo 1-1: *Walk along, and as you walk pay attention to your right hip. Does it move forward?*

each person. The major motion of the hip is forward, though, and this is the motion that you should direct your attention to. When you can easily identify the motion of the hip, continue walking for a few minutes and let the feeling sink into your body, so that you have a solid feel for just what the motion is.

Now, while you walk, direct your attention to the sensation of motion in your right shoulder. What does the right shoulder do as the right foot moves forward to take a step? Does it move forward or backward? (Photo 1-2)

To feel this motion, begin by thinking about your right hand. When the right foot goes forward, what does the right hand do? When you can feel the motion of the hand, let your attention move up your arm to your elbow and then on up to your shoulder. By doing this you should feel that as the right foot moves forward, the right shoulder moves backward. Walk some more and pay careful attention to the right hip and shoulder, noticing how the hip moves forward and the shoulder moves backward as the right foot moves forward to take a step.

When you have a good feeling for this hip and shoulder motion, try to exaggerate it. As the right foot moves forward to take a step, swing the right hip forward and the right shoulder backward much more than they

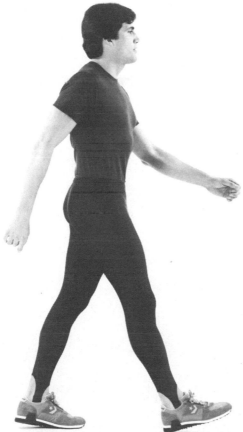

Photo 1-2: *Walk along, and now notice the right shoulder. What does it do when the right foot moves forward?*

would usually move. Then, as the left foot moves forward, reverse the motion of the right hip and shoulder so that the right shoulder moves far forward and the right hip moves far backward. Walk along for a few minutes like this, paying careful attention to the motion of the right hip and shoulder. (Photo 1-3)

Now try something different. Lock the right hip and shoulder together so that they do not move independently of one another as you walk. You will find that you have to move the whole right side of your body forward as you take a step with the right foot. To make this move easier, hold your right arm straight down alongside your body

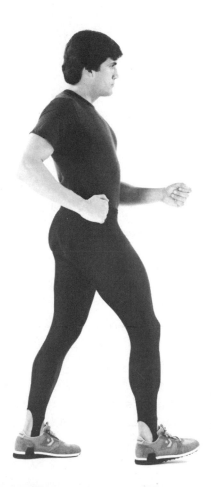

Photo 1-3: *Exaggerate the natural motion of your hip and shoulder as you walk.*

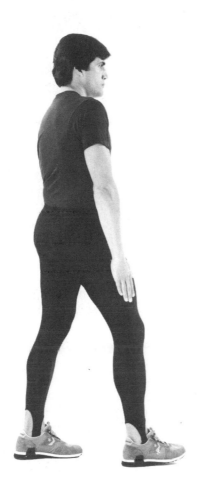

Photo 1-4: *Now lock your right hip and shoulder together as you walk; you'll probably find this awkward.*

with the palm of the hand on the right thigh. As you move, think about moving the whole right arm forward and letting the shoulder, ribs, and hip on that side move forward along with the arm. Once you can feel the motion, relax the right arm and let it swing easily as you walk. (Photo 1-4)

You will probably feel right away that this is an awkward and tiring way to walk, but try it out for a few minutes just to get the feel of this particular kind of walking. As you walk, look down at your feet and notice how locking the hip and shoulder together like this makes the feet come down on the ground in a clumsy, inefficient manner.

After a few minutes of walking with the hip and shoulder locked together, go back and walk again with the exaggerated hip and shoulder motion you tried earlier, letting the right hip swing far forward and the right shoulder swing far backward as the right foot moves forward to take a step. Does this motion feel easier and smoother after moving with the hip and shoulder locked together?

Now walk in your usual manner, without making any special adjustments, and think again about your right hip and shoulder. Can you feel exactly how the right hip and shoulder move when the right foot steps forward?

Stop walking, close your eyes, and just feel your whole body, comparing the left and right sides. Can you sense a difference between the side you've been paying attention to and the side you've ignored until now? Which foot takes more of your weight?

Stop and rest for a minute and then try this whole sequence of movements on the *left* side, noticing the motion of the left hip and shoulder when the left foot moves forward to take a step. Take plenty of time to work with each motion. Begin by noticing the motion of the left hip as the left foot moves forward to take a step. After a little of this, direct your attention to the left shoulder. Then try exaggerating the motion of the hip and shoulder, and then experiment with locking the left hip and shoulder together so that they do not move independently of one another as you walk. Can you find some differences between the motion of the left side of your body and the right side?

Again stop and rest for a couple of minutes. Resume walking, but now pay attention to the *left* shoulder and *right* hip as the right foot moves forward to take a step. Can you feel that the left shoulder and right hip both move forward together as the right foot moves forward? Think about the right shoulder and left hip as the left foot moves forward. Spend a few minutes working on both of these movements until you can easily feel the relative motion of the hips and shoulders as you walk. Do you find that shifting your attention around from one part of your body to the other as you walk changes the way you walk?

Continue walking and now exaggerate the normal movement of both hips and both shoulders. Walk like this for a few minutes, letting your attention move through your body. Then lock the hips and shoulders together on both sides and walk a little farther. Did you find that you hold your breath as you do this? Go back to the exaggerated movement of the hips and shoulders. Can you feel that as the hips rotate to the left, the shoulders rotate to the right, and as the hips rotate to the right, the shoulders rotate to the left?

Stop walking and stand still. How does your body feel? Is your breathing easier? Check your posture. Are you standing straighter?

After you've spent about an hour exploring the motion of your body while walking, sit down and spend a few minutes thinking about what you just did and what you could or couldn't feel as you were moving. All the movements that you made were fairly simple, and yet many people have a difficult time performing them. Changing the way you run means changing the way you move the different parts of your body; if you find these movements difficult while walking along slowly, how much more difficult will they be while running?

Our inability to perform these simple motions reflects a kind of blind spot in our awareness of ourselves. Most people find it difficult to pay attention to what they really are doing as they move. They have almost no feeling for what is going on in the central parts of their bodies—the hips, spine, and shoulders.

Imagine trying to draw a picture while blindfolded or trying to compose a piece of music while wearing earplugs. In most circumstances, what kind of results do you think you would get? Certainly nothing to get excited about. And yet this is exactly what we do when we try to run without an awareness of how all the different parts of the body move, and how the motion of each part affects all the others.

As long as we are wearing this "blindfold" over our bodies, all efforts to improve our running will be misdirected and there will be no real improvement. If, however, we can shed this blindfold and begin to explore body movement a little at a time, we will find new vistas of motion opening up on a daily basis and our running will improve beyond what we now imagine to be possible.

In subsequent chapters, we will explore these neglected body movements and the connections between them. We'll discover that as we become more aware of these parts, our walking and running will continue to improve, becoming easier, smoother, and more powerful.

Rich: The Beginnings of Awareness

The figure lumbering across the park reminded me of a B-movie Frankenstein monster. His whole upper body stiffened as he ran. From his hips to his head, I detected hardly a trace of relative motion in any of his body parts. This was Rich, 38 years old and one of my students—and a terrible runner.

But dedicated. Several years earlier he'd decided to "get in shape," and so he started running, probably because it was cheaper than buying a health-club membership. Unfortunately, whenever he ran more than a half-mile, his ankles, knees, and hips, not to mention the small of his back, hurt so much that the next morning he could barely get out of bed. It wasn't too surprising that he had abandoned running.

What I saw, watching Rich run that day, explained why running had proven such an obstacle for him. I had asked him to jog about 100 feet and then turn and sprint back as fast as he could. While sprinting, he exaggerated the stiffness of his upper body and complicated it by pulling his head down, almost freezing his upper chest. This effectively cut off his breathing. It also explained why his legs hurt so much: They were doing all the work, while the rest of his body seemed to be on permanent vacation.

When Rich stopped beside me, he was completely out of breath and gasping for air. A full minute passed before he could speak, and then he rested for several more minutes. All this, and he had only run 200 feet—less than the length of a football field! But perhaps I'm being too hard on the guy. He may well be superhuman: Can you run 200 feet holding your breath?

After he got his wind back, I asked Rich to walk along and pay attention to his right foot and hip. "What does your right hip do as your right foot moves forward to take a step?" I asked.

Rich looked at me like he thought I was crazy, so I repeated the question. Obviously, he just couldn't focus his attention on his foot and hip while he was moving. I figured that was the root of his problem: Rich seemed unaware of the fact that the movements of his foot and hip were inalienably connected.

I had him freeze with his right foot forward, as if he had stopped walking midstep. I told him to leave his feet on the ground where they were and to rotate his whole body left and right, and back and forth. When he was turning easily, I asked him to notice his right hip and to describe its motion to me.

When turning left and right while standing still like this, the hip makes a motion very similar to the motion that it makes while walking or running. However, when standing still we are not distracted by all the other movements that we have to make while walking or running, and it's easier to feel the motion of the hip.

After some concentration, Rich finally managed to determine that the right hip moved forward when he turned to the left and backward when he turned to the right. I had him spend several minutes doing this, focusing his attention on the right hip, then the right foot, then on the hip again, then on the right knee, back to the hip again, and so on.

We started to walk again. I asked him to think about what the right hip did as the right foot moved forward to take a step. This time it was a different story. Now he could feel the motion of his hip and it only took him a few minutes to connect it with the motion of his right foot.

He began walking very slowly and his face assumed a look of intense concentration. He slowed down even more. Suddenly, he came to a dead stop. "It moves forward," he said with amazement. "When my right foot moves forward, my right hip also moves forward. And I never felt it before now."

I had him walk some more and direct his attention to the motion of his right hip. I noticed that his walk had changed in a subtle but definite way and I asked him about it. He said that he could *feel* that he was walking differently but couldn't describe exactly what the difference was. It felt good, though, and now he could easily feel the motion of the right hip.

We continued with the exercise, working on the right shoulder and then spending some time on the left foot, hip, and shoulder. After about an hour of this we took a short rest, and then I asked Rich to repeat his initial run. He looked different this time. Not a lot, but enough to notice. He still tensed his upper body, which affected his breathing, so when he reached me he was again out of breath. But there was one big change: Through his gasps for air he said, with a big smile on his face, "My hips are moving. I can feel 'em."

In my teaching I have found that the worse someone runs, the less he can sense what is going on in his body. Likewise, the poorer the runner, the longer it takes him to develop this sense once he starts trying. Rich had a very difficult time feeling how his hips and shoulders moved when he walked. And this lack of feeling of how the parts of the body are moving is exactly the problem that many runners face when they try to improve.

Most runners, when attempting to improve, direct more effort to their feet and sometimes their knees. But they usually ignore their hips, spine, and shoulders. Only a small amount of improvement is possible by proceeding this way.

What most runners need is a change in the *way* they run—that is, a redirection of the effort of running into other parts of the body. And the first step in this process of redirection is developing an awareness of how these other parts of the body move. Once an awareness is established, the change is practically automatic, as Rich found out and I saw when he began to feel how his right hip moved as his right foot moved forward to take a step.

When this happens there is a new feeling of ease, and a sense of achievement as well. After a lesson like this, you always go away with a smile on your face, no matter how tired or sore you might be.

2

The Muscles of the Back

Stand up and with each hand reach around to the small of your back, just on either side of your spine, right above the pelvis. (Photo 2-1) Walk around a little and with your hands feel the muscles there. Notice how the muscles work as you walk.

These muscles in the lower back are some of the largest and strongest in the body. As you can clearly feel, they do something very distinct as you walk. Walk around some more, feeling these muscles. When the right foot moves forward, which one of these muscles contracts, the right or the left?

Lie down flat on your back on a carpeted surface with your legs stretched out straight, feet slightly apart. Notice how your pelvis and upper back (between the shoulder blades) lie flat on the floor. What about the small of the back, between the pelvis and the upper back, in the area that you just felt with your hands while walking? Is that part of your body touching the floor? It probably isn't. Reach under yourself with one hand and feel how far off the floor the spine is here.

14

Why is this area held up off the floor while the rest of the spine is not? Evidently, the muscles in this area must be contracting to raise the spine up. Think about what this means: For a muscle to perform a movement it must first be in a relaxed, lengthened state. A muscle that is already contracted is unable to do any work until it first relaxes and becomes longer. Only then is it able to contract again.

With most people, the lower spine is well up off the floor and the lower back muscles are strongly contracted *all the time,* even when they lie on their backs and "relax." This means that these muscles, among the most powerful in the body, are unable to do their proper share of the work during walking and running. As a result, we do not

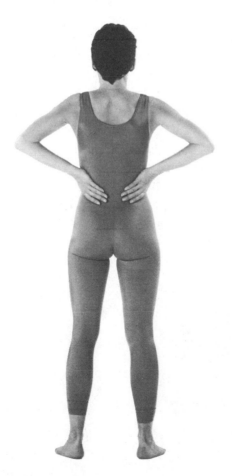

Photo 2-1: *Reach around and feel the large muscles on each side of the spine just above the pelvis.*

run as well or as powerfully as we might. And the other muscles in the body, which have to work even harder to compensate for the idle lower back muscles, become sore and more susceptible to injury. What we need to do, then, is lengthen these muscles so that they can do their proper share of the work when we run.

As you lie on your back, try to push the small of the back down flat onto the floor to lengthen the back muscles. What happens as you do this? You'll probably find that it's a big strain throughout your body and that you stiffen your chest and hold your breath. Do you think you could run well like this? Probably not.

A direct effort, then, probably won't flatten the back and lengthen the lower back muscles. Then how can we make these muscles become longer and so improve our running?

Still on your back, draw up your knees so that your feet are flat on the floor, fairly close to your buttocks, and a comfortable distance apart from each other. Again put one hand under your back and note how far off the floor the spine is now. You'll notice that the spine has moved down toward the floor a bit, lengthening the lower back muscles.

Leaving the hand where it is, slowly rock the pelvis up

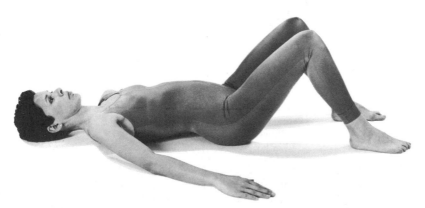

Photo 2-2: *Lie on your back and rock your pelvis up so that the small of your back comes up off the ground.*

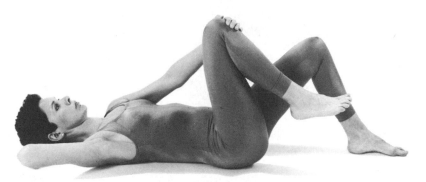

Photo 2-3: *Still on your back, place your right hand behind your head and your left hand below your right knee.*

a little so that the small of the back raises up off the floor a bit and the point of contact of the pelvis and floor rolls down toward the tailbone. Then relax, letting the small of the back come down. (Photo 2-2) Repeat this motion a few times, using your hand to feel how the back moves; then remove your hand and try to feel just how the spine moves up and down without the hand to help.

Now relax. Place the right hand behind the head, and with the left hand grasp the right leg just below the kneecap. The right foot will be up off the floor. The left knee is still bent and the left foot is resting flat on the floor. (Photo 2-3)

Very slowly raise the head and right hand, move the right elbow toward the right knee, and the right knee toward the right elbow. (Photo 2-4) Use the right hand to help lift the head and the left hand to help pull the right knee. Don't try to touch the knee to the elbow; just move them a few inches closer to each other, and then let the head and right hand and elbow move back to the floor and the right knee move back until it is supported by the left arm. Repeat the motion several times, slowly and without straining, and make sure that you are not holding your breath. Is it easier to breathe in or out as you move the right knee and elbow toward each other? Try both ways several times. Which feels easier?

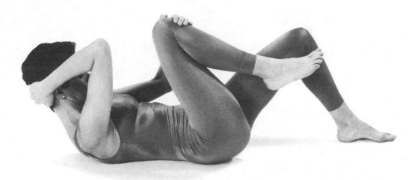

Photo 2-4: *Slowly move your right elbow toward your right knee and your right knee toward your right elbow.*

Continue to move the right knee and elbow toward each other and direct your attention to the back. Notice how the small of the back lengthens and presses down onto the floor as the knee and elbow approach each other, and then rises up as the knee and elbow move away.

Repeat this motion, moving the right knee and elbow toward each other about 25 times. Then stop, stretch your legs out straight on the floor, and rest both of your arms beside your body. Notice the relationship now between the small of the back and the floor. You will feel that the spine has lowered toward the floor a little, lengthening the lower back muscles.

Most of your effort was directed to the right side of the body. Can you feel that the right side has changed more than the left? With each hand, reach under the lower spine and feel the distance from the back to the floor. Is there a difference between the left and right sides? Can you feel it without your hands?

Again draw up your knees, feet flat on the floor, slightly apart, and close to your buttocks. Place the left hand behind the head, and with the right hand grasp the left leg just below the knee.

As before, move the left knee and elbow closer to each other, and then relax and let the head, hand, and elbow rest on the floor. Repeat the motion, moving slowly and without straining, and think about how your spine

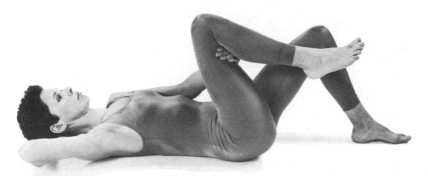

Photo 2-5: *This time place your right hand behind your head and left hand* behind *your right knee.*

moves against the floor. Notice your breathing and how the pelvis rolls a little on the floor. After about 25 repetitions, stretch out and rest. As you lie there, think about the small of the back. Do the left and right sides feel more equal now?

Again draw up the knees, feet flat on the floor. Place the right hand behind the head, and with the left hand grasp the right thigh just behind the knee so that the hand is held between the upper and lower leg. (Photo 2-5)

Again lift the head, move the right elbow toward the right knee, and the right knee toward the right elbow, helping with the left hand. (Photo 2-6) Move the elbow

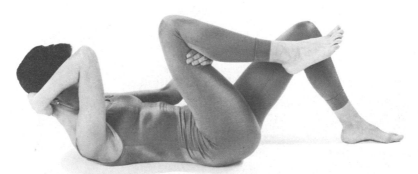

Photo 2-6: *Move your right elbow toward your right knee and vice versa. Can you feel your weight shift on the floor?*

and knee closer together and then let them move easily back to the floor. Repeat this move slowly, about 20 to 25 times, noticing how the spine curves against the floor and how the small of the back presses down as the elbow and knee come closer together. Can you feel how your weight shifts to one side on the floor as you do this?

Notice your breathing as you move. Do you hold your breath as you start to lift your head? Try breathing in as you lift a few times, then try breathing out. Which way is easier? Stop, stretch out, and rest, noticing how your body lies on the floor.

Draw your knees up as before. Place the left hand behind the head, and with the right hand grasp the left thigh just behind the knee so that the hand is held between the upper and lower leg. Slowly move the left elbow toward the left knee and the knee toward the elbow. Let the head and elbow return to the floor and the left knee move back; repeat this motion about 25 times. To which side of the body does the weight shift now? Stretch out and rest.

Check the way that your body lies on the floor now. Is the small of the back resting closer to the floor?

Again draw up your knees. Place the right hand behind the head, and with the left hand grasp the left leg just below the kneecap. (Photo 2-7)

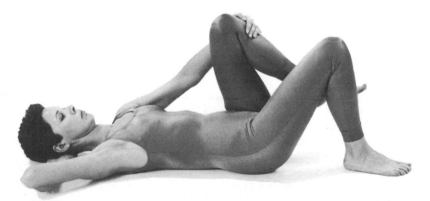

Photo 2-7: *This time, place your right hand behind your head and your left hand below your* left *knee.*

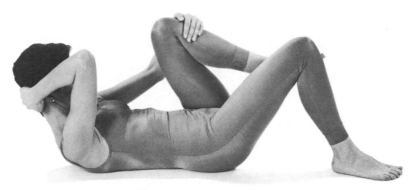

Photo 2-8: *Now move your right elbow toward your left knee and your left knee toward your right elbow.*

Now direct the right elbow toward the left knee, moving slowly, and notice how your back moves against the floor. (Photo 2-8) In the previous motions all of the work was on either the right or the left side. In this move the right side of the upper body and the left side of the lower body are doing the work. Notice how you can feel this in the way your back moves against the floor. Repeat the motion about 25 times, then stretch out and rest.

Again draw up the knees, feet flat on the floor. Place the left hand behind the head, and with the right hand grasp the right leg just below the kneecap. Move the left elbow toward the right knee just a bit and then let the knee and elbow move back down toward the floor. Repeat the motion about 25 times. Notice how the movement becomes easier and the knee and elbow come closer each time without straining, as you think about your spine, your pelvis, and your breathing—in short, your whole body. Stretch out and rest a little. How does the small of the back feel now?

Again draw up your knees. Interlace your fingers and place the backs of your hands on the floor under your head so that your head rests snugly in the cup formed by your hands. (Photo 2-9) Moving very slowly and using your hands for support, lift your head up as if you were going to look at your feet. Notice how the elbows come closer together as the head rises, and how your spine

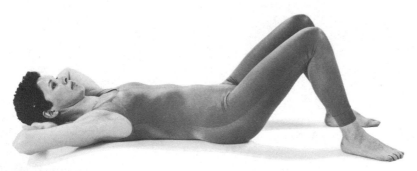

Photo 2-9: *Lie on your back with your feet flat on the floor and interlace your fingers behind your head.*

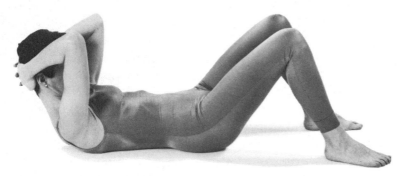

Photo 2-10: *Lift your head up, bringing your elbows closer together; pay attention to your spine as you do this.*

feels. (Photo 2-10) Lower the head to the floor and repeat the motion. Keep your feet flat on the floor.

As you risc up, pay careful attention to the spine. Notice how, as the head lifts, the vertebrae of the upper spine come up off the floor one by one. See if you can feel each vertebra as it comes up when you lift the head and hands, and then as it comes back to the floor as you lower the head and hands.

Continue moving like this and notice the small of the back. Notice how the vertebrae move down to the floor as the head and hands come up. Can you discover a connection between the motion of the vertebrae in the lower back and the upper back? Make sure that you don't hold your breath as you do this. Stop moving for a minute and rest as you are, feet flat on the floor and hands behind your head.

Now, very slowly tilt the pelvis, raise the small of the back up off the floor a little, and then let it back down. Repeat this motion about five or six times; as you let the small of the back down, continue the motion of the spine downward and use this motion to help lift the head and hands. Then lower the head and hands to the floor. Again lift the lower spine up a little and then press it down to the floor, lifting the head as you do so.

Notice how easily the head lifts when the lower back gets involved in the motion. Repeat this motion several more times, then stretch out and rest. Check the small of the back. You will feel that it is even closer to the floor and has become even longer. Continue to lie still and rest for a minute or so, letting your attention wander up and down your spine.

Again draw up your knees. With the left hand grasp the right leg just below the kneecap. With the right hand grasp the bottom of the right foot from the outside. If this is a strain, grasp the right ankle. (Photo 2-11) Move the

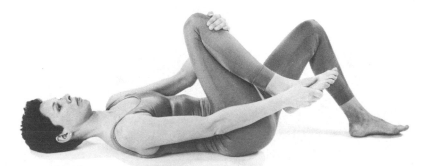

Photo 2-11: *Now grab your right foot with your right hand, and with your left hand hold your right leg just below the knee.*

right knee toward the forehead and move the forehead toward the knee. (Photo 2-12)

Reverse the motion, lowering the head to the floor, and then repeat. As you move, don't strain to touch your head to your knee; just move as far as is comfortable and no more. If you work and strain you will be defeating the purpose of the movements, which is to improve the way that you move—more specifically, the *quality* of the movement. Repeat the motion 20 or more times and then stretch out and rest.

Draw up your knees again. With the right hand, grasp the left leg below the kneecap, and with the left

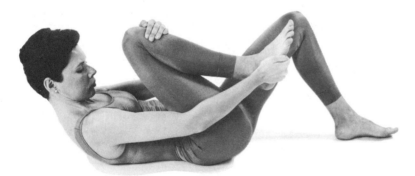

Photo 2-12: *Move your forehead and knee toward each other simultaneously; move only as far as is easy.*

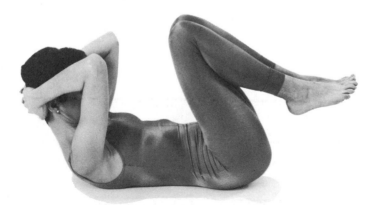

Photo 2-13: *With your hands behind your head, lift your head and move your knees and elbows closer together.*

hand, grasp the bottom of the left foot from the outside. As before, move the forehead and knee closer to each other and then farther away. Do this 20 to 25 times and then stop and rest, arms and legs stretched out on the floor.

Interlace the fingers behind the head and draw up the knees. Lift the head, arms, and both legs so that the knees and elbows approach each other. (Photo 2-13) Holding the knees and elbows close together, rock the body up and down from the head to the pelvis so that the spine moves on the floor like the rocker on a rocking chair. Bring your feet and legs back over your head to rock

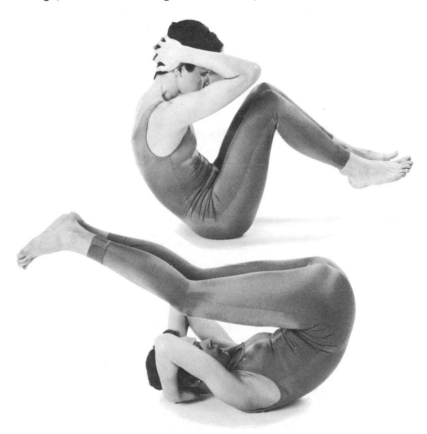

Photos 2-14, 2-15: *Holding your knees and elbows close together, roll up and down along your spine. Is the motion smooth, or are there flat, bumpy spots?*

back, and forward toward your buttocks to rock forward. (Photos 2-14, 2-15) Is the whole spine evenly curved so that the rocking motion is smooth and even, or are there flat, bumpy spots? Rock up and down for a while, then stop, stretch out your arms and legs, and rest.

Notice how your body lies on the floor; pay particular attention to the spine and the small of the back. You should be able to feel clearly where the spine is located and how the small of your back is much flatter against the floor.

In a normal—not *average*—body, the small of the back will not lie perfectly flat; instead, it will be lifted up just a little. A completely flat lower back would cause problems in movement, just as one with an excessive curvature does.

By moving slowly and easily as you just did and paying attention to what you are doing, you can help the spine to move toward its optimal position, neither too flat nor too curved. This is very different from the way we typically learn movement, by figuring out in advance what we want to do and then trying to force our bodies into some posture or pattern of movement that may not be right for us.

Very slowly, taking at least a full 60 seconds, roll over to one side, come up onto your hands and knees, and then stand up. As you stand up, think about the small of the back. Do you contract the muscles there as you stand?

Reach around and feel the small of the back with your hands. Walk around a little. Is the feeling clearer now than when you first tried to feel this area? What can you feel without your hands?

Walk around some more and try swinging your hips and shoulders in the exaggerated way suggested in the previous chapter. Do the hips move a little farther? A little more easily? How do you think this improvement in the motion of the hips will affect your running?

The next time you run, start off slowly and pay attention to the small of your back. If you move carefully you may be able to avoid contracting the back muscles unnecessarily, and your running will improve in a way that you have never felt before.

In the next chapter we will explore how the lower back muscles connect to the shoulders and neck, and you will make further improvements. But don't try this right away. Give your body at least one day, preferably two, to let the changes produced as a result of what you just did sink in and become integrated into your own way of moving.

Bif: Running and Breathing

At 28, Bif had developed into a serious amateur runner, averaging about 50 miles a week. He had run in a few races and done well, but like most runners, he was sure that he could do better. So he decided to try my running class.

After several sessions Bif's running started to change. About that time he mentioned that his breathing had changed somehow.

"I don't know whether I'm running better or worse now," he said, frustrated. "For instance, even though it seems like I have more wind, I feel short of breath at the same time. Now explain that to me."

I asked Bif to hold his hands up in front of himself and interlace his fingers. "Which thumb is on top?" I asked.

Bif looked at me suspiciously. "What's that got to do with running?" he asked.

"Just try it," I said. "I want to show you something."

Bif interlaced his fingers and looked down at them. "The left thumb is on top," he said.

"Now," I said, "cross them again, but this time change the interlacing so that the right thumb is on top." He did this and I asked if he felt anything.

"Sure I do," he said. "It feels different."

"Wrong?" I inquired.

"Yeah, it feels wrong. So what's the point?" he asked as he dropped his hands.

"Well, is it really wrong, or just different?" I continued.

"It's not wrong, I guess, but it sure feels wrong,"
Bif replied.

"That's what's going on with your breathing," I said.
"Just because it's different now from the way that you
usually breathe, it feels wrong. But it's not wrong, any
more than your hands were wrong. It's just different, and
probably better.

"Changing your breathing is very tricky business," I
continued, "because a change in breathing always involves
a change in posture and movement as well. You don't
suddenly change the way you breathe and *only* the way
you breathe; you actually modify your whole body.
Sometimes the new way of breathing will feel 'wrong'—the
way your hands felt wrong—because you have changed an
old, familiar habit. Most likely, your breathing is better and
easier now than ever before. This slight disorientation that
you think of as discomfort will pass soon."

"I don't know," Bif protested. "Better breathing ought
to *feel* better. How can I be absolutely sure that what's
happened is good for me and for my running?"

As we continued to talk, he told me about his dog,
Nicky. When Bif ran, Nicky liked to run with him. Usually
the dog had a good time, scampering far ahead of Bif,
then running back or off to the side to examine something
interesting. Yet after a run, Nicky would be as fresh as if
he had just awakened from a nap, while Bif himself would
be out of breath. Bif had always marveled at the dog's
boundless energy.

Over the last few weeks, however, a very strange
thing had begun to happen. Nicky, it seemed, was having
an increasingly difficult time keeping up with Bif. He was
not running out in front so much, and hardly ever ran off
to the side any more. And at the end of the run, Nicky now
appeared to be getting a little winded.

In fact, during the last three or four runs, the
situation had become critical. Bif would arrive back home
at the end of a 7- to 10-mile run almost as fresh as when
he started. Nicky, however, could barely make it through
the last mile, and upon arriving at home the dog would
collapse on the ground, completely exhausted.

"You know," Bif said to me, "I'm going to have to start leaving Nicky at home."

I asked him what he made of the situation. Bif thought it over and decided that either he himself was running a lot faster and breathing more easily or his dog was ill. Since the dog was as healthy as ever the rest of the time, Bif finally was forced to admit that his running and breathing were improving, even though he didn't feel like they were. But he still couldn't believe that he could run so much better and faster and not feel it.

I pointed out to him that this was a common problem for many people trying to improve their running. That is, better running doesn't *feel* like better running to them. In fact, it may even feel "wrong," just as the unfamiliar way of interlacing the fingers feels wrong. Thus, even when they improve a little, they don't notice the difference or they feel uncomfortable with the change. So they soon slip back into their old, inefficient habits. When someone starts using all the different parts of his body during running, he actually begins to run faster and with less effort, and to breathe more easily. Yet even then he may not realize how much he has improved, unless he pays careful attention to his body and to what's going on around him.

Most of Bif's running problems are gone, but now he has a different kind of problem. If he takes Nicky out to run, the poor animal nearly has a heart attack trying to keep up. On the other hand, if he leaves Nicky at home, the dog feels neglected and sulks around the rest of the evening. It is, indeed, a difficult problem. If you're going to have a problem with your running, however, I suppose this is the kind of problem to have.

3

Connections in the Back

Most of the connections between our hips and shoulders that cause them to move properly when we are walking and running operate through the muscles of the back. For most of us, the back is a rather cloudy area in our awareness. We don't usually pay too much attention to what goes on there unless we develop a backache. However, the old expression "Put your back into it," heard whenever someone is required to make an extraordinary effort, shows that we recognize the back muscles as a source of strength and power.

In the previous chapter you discovered how the large muscles of the lower back work as you walk and run, and how the work of these muscles can be improved by gently exploring the connections between the muscles of the front and the back of the body. In this chapter we will explore how the muscles of the lower back and hips connect to the muscles of the upper back, neck, and shoulders. As these connections get clearer, you will feel a kind of balance in your running that wasn't there before. This balance comes from having the muscles of the neck, shoulders, and upper back work in a more harmonious way with the muscles of the lower back and hips.

To begin this exploration, lie down on your stomach and turn your face to the left. Place the palm of your left hand on the floor under your head, place the palm of your right hand on the back of your left hand, and rest your right ear on the back of your right hand. (Photo 3-1)

Very slowly lift the head and the right arm up off the floor a little and then set them back down. (Photo 3-2) You needn't raise them more than a half-inch. Repeat the motion, moving slowly, and make sure that the whole right arm—the hand, elbow, and shoulder—comes up off the floor, and that the back of the right hand continues to touch the right ear.

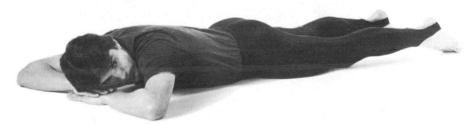

Photo 3-1: *On your stomach, place your right hand on your left, palms down, and rest your right ear on your hands.*

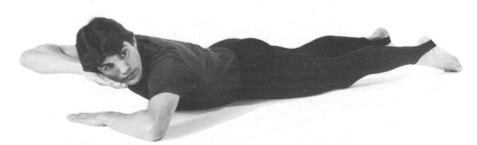

Photo 3-2: *Lift your head and right arm up off the floor a little and then set them back down.*

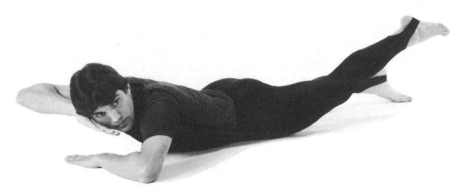

Photo 3-3: *Lift the head and right arm again, and also lift the left leg off the floor.*

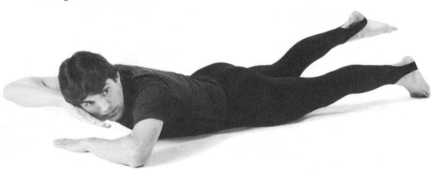

Photo 3-4: *Now switch legs so that you're lifting your head, right arm, and* right *leg.*

Repeat the motion slowly about 10 times and then stop and rest for a minute. Now lift the head and right arm again, and also lift the left leg, keeping the knee straight. (Photo 3-3) Repeat this motion, lifting the head, right arm, and left leg, and notice how the center of the body pushes into the floor as the arm, leg, and head lift up.

Try this move about 10 times and then switch legs, so that you lift the head, right arm, and right leg. (Photo 3-4) Try this move about 10 times, too, and then stop and rest.

Think about what you just did. Was it easier to lift one leg than to lift the other? Lift the head and right arm as before and experiment with the legs, lifting the right leg a few times, then the left leg, then the right, and so on. Which leg and hip connect to the neck and right shoulder in a way that makes one leg easier to lift than the other?

You may not be able to feel this clearly at first, because you aren't used to paying attention to small details of motion like this. Attention to these small details, however, is what makes the difference between a good runner and a poor one. By making small, slow, easy motions as you just did, and paying careful attention to how the whole body is involved in the motion, you will increase your ability to feel these differences, and your control will improve.

Again lift the head, right arm, and left leg and then lower them slowly back to the floor. Repeat the motion about 25 times and as you move, let your attention wander around your body. Can you feel your weight shift on the floor as you lift up? What about your breathing? Do you hold your breath as you move or is your breathing slow and easy? Think about your spine and shoulder blades. How do they move—or do they move at all—as you lift the head, right arm, and left leg? Lower everything to the floor and rest briefly on your stomach.

Very slowly lift your head, turn it to face right, and reverse your hands so that the left hand is on top. Now your left ear rests on the back of your left hand, and the palm of the left hand rests on the back of the right hand, which is on the floor.

Slowly lift the head and left hand, making sure that the left shoulder, elbow, and hand all come up off the floor, and that the right arm stays on the floor. Raise them only as far as is easy and then lower the head and left arm back down. Repeat the motion about 10 times and then rest.

Now lift the head and left arm together, and also lift the right leg off the floor just a little. As these parts rise, make sure that the knee and the foot both come up off the floor. Raise them up as far as is easy and then go back to the floor. Repeat the motion about 10 times and then try it while you raise the left leg.

Stop and rest. As you lie there, think about what you just did. Did one leg feel easier to lift than the other? Again lift the head and left arm and experiment with the legs, lifting first the right leg a few times, then the left, then the right, and so on. Follow that with a rest.

Lift the head and left arm as before, and also lift the right leg. Lift them up only as far as is easy, then lower them back to the floor. Repeat the motion about 25 times. As you move, direct your attention to the different parts of your body, as before. Notice how your weight shifts on the floor and how you breathe. Stop, roll over onto your back, and rest.

As you lie there, think about the spine. How does it lie against the floor? In particular, notice the small of the back. Is it raised up off the floor even more than usual? You will almost certainly feel that the small of the back is up off the floor. This is caused by the residual contraction of the back muscles, which have been working to lift the head, arms, and legs.

Draw your knees up so that the feet are flat on the floor near your buttocks and interlace your fingers behind your head. (Photo 3-5) Slowly raise the head up, helping with the hands, and let the elbows come closer together. (Photo 3-6) Raise the head up as far as is easy and then lower it back down to the floor. Repeat the motion about 10 or 15 times and then stretch out and rest.

Notice how the small of the back has lowered toward the floor. Lie still and rest for a minute. As you lie there, scan your body, noticing how it makes contact with the floor. Do the left and right sides seem to lay equally against the floor?

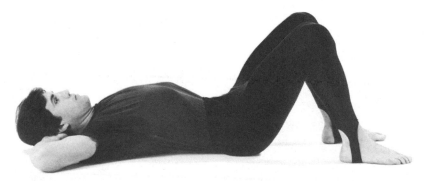

Photo 3-5: *Now draw your knees up, feet flat on the floor, and interlace your fingers behind your head.*

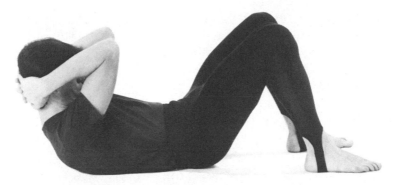

Photo 3-6: *Raise your head, bringing your elbows together; go only as far as is easy, then lower back to the floor.*

Turn and lie on your stomach with your face turned to the left, the right ear resting on the back of the right hand, and the palm of the right hand resting on the back of the left hand. Slowly raise the head, right arm and hand, and left leg a little way off the floor, and then let them go back. Make sure that the *whole* right arm—the hand, forearm, and elbow—comes up off the floor and that the right ear continues to touch the back of the right hand.

Continue to raise and lower the head, right arm, and left leg, and now flex the left ankle so that as the foot comes down, the bottom of the toes and the ball of the foot come in contact with the floor. (Photo 3-7) Repeat the motion about 25 times and then stop and rest, lying on your stomach.

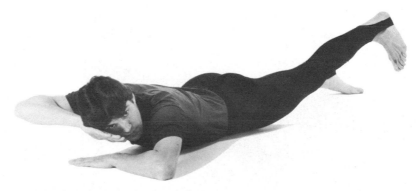

Photo 3-7: *Continue to raise and lower the head, right arm, and left leg, and now flex the left ankle.*

Now slowly turn your head to face right and change your hands over so that the left hand is on top. The left ear is resting on the back of the left hand. Flex your right foot so that the bottom of the toes and the ball of the foot touch the floor.

Raise your head, left arm, and right leg up as far as is easy and then lower them. Repeat the motion about 25 times. As you move, pay attention to the different parts of your body. Notice how the spine moves in back and how the stomach presses down into the floor. Notice your breathing. Is it smooth and easy? When you have finished, turn and lie on your back and rest.

As you lie there, scan your body and notice which parts touch the floor. Are some areas higher up off the floor than before? Have other areas lowered closer to the floor?

Turn and lie on your stomach. Place the right hand on top of the left hand and rest the forehead on the back of

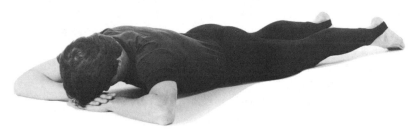

Photo 3-8: *Lie on your stomach; rest your forehead on the back of your right hand and your right hand on top of your left.*

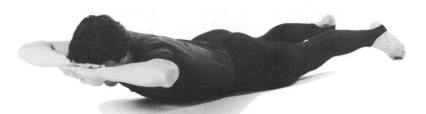

Photo 3-9: *Raise your head and both arms off the floor; make sure your forehead maintains contact with your hand.*

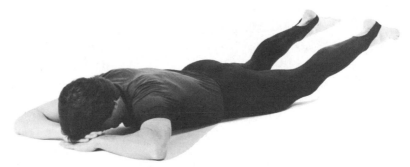

Photo 3-10: *Lift your feet and knees off the floor a little and then lower them; notice your head and hands as you lift.*

the right hand. (Photo 3-8) From this position, raise the head and both arms off the floor a little. (Photo 3-9) Make sure that the forehead continues to touch the back of the right hand and that both elbows lift up along with the head. Then lower everything back to the floor.

Repeat this move slowly about 10 times and notice your knees and feet. What do the knees and feet do as the head and arms rise? If you move slowly and pay attention, you should be able to feel that the feet and knees rise up off the floor a little as the head and arms come up.

Stop and rest briefly, then lift the feet and knees off the floor a little, keeping the knees straight. (Photo 3-10) Lower the feet and knees and repeat the lifting motion. As you move the legs, notice the head and hands. Do they tend to lift up a little as the legs rise? Continue to move slowly, lifting the legs, and notice how the upper body moves as the legs rise.

Stop moving and rest, lying on your stomach. Think about the movements you just made. The upper and lower ends of the body were raised up into the air, and so the middle of the body, the abdominal area, must have been pressed more into the floor. Did you notice the increase of pressure in that area as you lifted the head, arms, and legs?

Now raise the head, arms, and both legs a little, and pay careful attention to the point of contact between the center of the body—the stomach—and the floor. (Photo 3-11) Notice how the stomach must press down into the floor if the two ends of the body are to be lifted. Let everything back down onto the floor, and then repeat this motion, going up and down, about 15 times.

Now, instead of thinking about lifting the head, arms, and legs, concentrate on pushing your abdomen into the floor. Try this move and notice what happens. The head, arms, and legs lift almost as before, but you may feel that the lifting motion is easier when you think about pushing the stomach down into the floor. Continue to push the stomach down into the floor and notice how the top part of the body balances the bottom part as they both rise up. After about 10 or 15 movements, stop and rest.

Raise the head and both arms and legs two or three times. Notice the amount of effort and the range of motion. Do you feel that this movement has become easier as a result of pushing the stomach down as you raise the head and legs?

Raise the head, arms, and legs again, and hold. From this position, move the eyes to look up toward your forehead and then down in the direction of the floor. Move the eyes up and down about 10 times, making sure that you do not hold your breath, and then rest on the floor on your stomach.

Once more lift the head, arms, and legs and notice the range of motion and the amount of effort. Did the motion of the eyes make a further difference in the

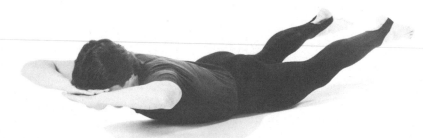

Photo 3-11: *Now raise your head, arms, and both legs a little; pay attention to your stomach as it touches the floor.*

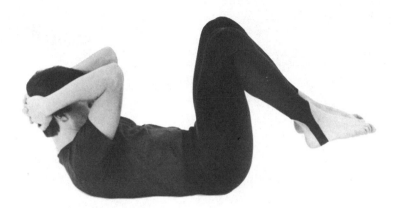

Photo 3-12: *On your back, with your knees up and your fingers interlaced behind your head, move your knees and elbows closer together.*

movement? Turn and lie on your back and rest. As you lie there, notice your spine in relation to the floor. Is the lower spine touching the floor?

Draw up your knees to set your feet flat on the floor and interlace your fingers behind your head. Move the knees and elbows closer together, raising your head and feet and folding your body, and then let the head, hands, and feet come back to the floor. (Photo 3-12) Repeat the move about 20 times, letting yourself breathe out as you fold the body, and notice how the spine presses against the floor. Stop moving, stretch out, and rest. Check your lower back. Is it closer to the floor now?

After a minute or two of resting on your back, turn and lie on your stomach one more time. Turn your face to the left and rest the right ear on the back of the right hand. Place the palm of the right hand on the back of the left and flex both feet so that the bottoms of the toes and the balls of the feet touch the floor. (Photo 3-13)

Slowly lift the head, right arm, and left leg, then lower them back to the floor. Turn the head to the right and reverse the hands so that the left ear rests on the back of the left hand. Lift the head, left arm, and right leg, then lower them back to the floor. Turn the head to face left and

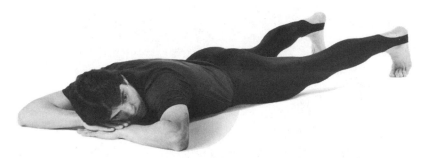

Photo 3-13: *On your stomach, rest your head on your right hand and flex both feet so the balls of your feet touch the floor.*

again reverse the hands so that the right hand is on top. Once again raise the head, right arm, and left leg, and lower them to the floor. Turn the head to face the other way, reverse the hands, and lift again, and so on.

As you move like this, you will find that with each move you lift one shoulder and arm and the opposite hip and thigh, and that the head faces the leg being lifted. On the next move, the other shoulder, arm, hip, and thigh come up, and so on.

Repeat this move about 25 times and notice how the raising of one shoulder connects through the muscles of the back to cause the opposite hip and leg to rise. If you were standing, the motion of the shoulders and back would help to move the legs backward—that is, they would increase the power of your walking or running. If someone were to raise you straight up to standing and you continued to move just as you are, you would walk along the floor. Stop moving, turn and lie on your back, and rest.

As you lie there, mentally review these movements. The motions of the body were very similar to the motions of walking, except that you were lying on your stomach instead of standing up. When you are lying on your stomach, gravity acts on your body from a different direction and causes your back muscles to react in unusual ways. In this position you can feel the connections between the hips and shoulders clearly, because the back muscles must work directly against gravity, and the proper parts of the body must lift to balance the effort.

Draw up your knees, roll over to one side, and stand up. Walk around a little and experiment with the motion of the hips and shoulders as you are aware of them now. Notice the feeling of power and ease that comes from having a clear sensation of how the back muscles work to organize the movements of the hips and shoulders.

Rod: The Problem in the Knee Is in the Shoulder

In the first hour of one of my recent running classes, about a dozen people were walking around in a large circle. I had asked them at first to pay attention to their right hips as their right feet moved forward to take a step. After everyone had learned to feel the right hip moving forward when the right foot stepped forward, I asked them to feel the motion of their right shoulders. When everyone could feel how the right shoulder moved backward as the right foot moved forward, I asked them first to exaggerate the relative motions of the right hip and shoulder, and then to lock the hip and shoulder together, walk that way, and notice what it felt like.

After a dozen steps with the hip and shoulder locked together, one of the students, Rod, suddenly winced and stopped walking. "Boy," he said, "that really hurts my right knee."

He looked discouraged and I asked him what was the matter. "Well, every time I do any serious running," he said, "my right knee goes to pot and I have to stop. Looks like it's not going to be any different here."

"How did your knee feel just a minute ago when you were exaggerating the motion of the hip and shoulder?" I asked him.

"Well, it felt OK, I guess. It must not have been hurting, since I didn't really notice it."

"All right, go back to that exaggerated movement of the hip and shoulder and see how the knee feels."

Rod stepped out, swinging his hip and shoulder as he walked along. He walked once around the room with a growing look of disbelief on his face. "It almost doesn't hurt at all," he said. "I can hardly feel any pain."

"Now try walking with your hip and shoulder locked together again," I told him.

Cautiously, Rod began to walk, his hip and shoulder locked together. After a few steps he winced again and stopped. "The pain's back," he said.

"So what does that tell you?" I asked.

Rod thought about my question for a while. Finally he said, "Since my knee hurts when I move the hip and shoulder together, and since it doesn't hurt when I move them in opposite directions, it must be something in the motion of the hip and shoulder that causes the knee to hurt." He paused. "But how can the shoulder affect the knee like that?" he asked.

"That's a tricky question to answer," I said, "and it's probably a slightly different answer for each person. But this is what usually happens. Whether walking or running, every time you take a step, the whole weight of your body comes down on your knee. For efficient use of the knee, your weight should come down in such a way that it is distributed equally over the whole knee joint.

"If, for example, the weight comes down more on the inside of the knee, the cartilage there can start to deteriorate and the tendons on the outside of the joint may get stretched and become prone to injury. If you don't do any serious running, you may never notice any problem with your knee. But if you start a tough work-out schedule or injure your knee slightly, it could give you trouble.

"The important thing to notice is that the problem in the knee usually doesn't originate in the knee itself, but instead comes from a misuse somewhere else in the body. You could say that the problem in the knee is actually in the shoulder. Or sometimes it's in the neck, or the spine, or even the eyes.

"In other words, the exact position of the knee as it assumes the weight of the body is not determined by the knee itself, but by the hips, spine, shoulders, and head."

Rod and most of the rest of my students thought this sounded reasonable, but a few people weren't completely convinced. So I asked the class to walk some more and really exaggerate the motion of the hip and shoulder. When they were all doing this, I told them to look down and notice how their feet hit the floor. They all quickly saw that their feet were coming down on the floor one in front of the other. With a few people, the feet actually crossed over each other so that the right foot hit the floor just to the left of where the left foot hit, and vice versa.

Then I asked the students to lock their hips and shoulders together and watch their feet. They saw that their feet came down on the floor wide apart.

In the first case, as you exaggerate the motion of the hip and shoulder, the weight of the body shifts to the outside of the leg; therefore, the weight comes down on the outside of the knee. In the second case, with the shoulder and hip locked together, the weight shifts to the inside of the leg and so comes down on the inside of the knee. Somewhere between these extremes there is a movement, a balanced movement, where the weight comes down on the knee just right. By exploring the two extremes like this, we can find that middle ground where the knee works perfectly.

"There's even more to it than that," I told the class. "Lock your hips and shoulders together again and walk. Notice how your heels bang down onto the floor."

Everyone started to walk and I could tell what they were doing even with my eyes closed. That kind of walking makes a lot of noise. You can almost hear the knee cartilage disintegrating.

"OK," I said, "now just walk naturally and be sure to let your hips and shoulders swing easily." Immediately, the noise level in the room dropped dramatically.

"Do you think that banging your heels into the floor like that will build strong ankles and knees?" I asked softly. Nobody even bothered to answer my question, but I could see the answer that I wanted in Rod's face. There wasn't a trace of pain there.

4

The Hips Alone

The hips are the powerhouse of the entire body. The muscles around the hips, as well as in the thighs and lower back, are the largest and strongest you have. Despite this, many people have very little feeling for what goes on in their hips. In my classes I continually find people who say with utmost confidence that one hip is moving forward, while I and everyone else can see clearly that it is moving backward. When this situation prevails during walking or running, a person wastes the power of the hips through misdirection. Power is useless without control, and control is impossible without awareness.

In this lesson you will explore the motion of the hips; in order to do this, you'll be lying on one side. When lying on your side, you're free to move one hip in various directions as slowly as you wish. This way you can find out if you are actually moving the hip in the direction you *think* you're moving it. When standing—and especially when running—it's much more difficult to do this.

As your awareness of your hips' movements increases, you will have better control of the power of your hips. The

44

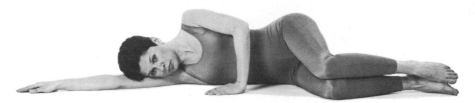

Photo 4-1: *Lie on your right side and bend your knees and hips at right angles; rest your head on your right arm and place the left hand on the floor in front of your chest.*

result will be a surprising increase in the power of your running and, in fact, in the power of all your movements.

Lie on your right side with your knees and hips bent at right angles as if you were sitting upright in a chair. Stretch your right arm out comfortably on the floor overhead and rest your right ear on your arm. Rest the palm of the left hand on the floor just in front of your chest. The left knee should be on top of the right knee and the left ankle should be on top of the right ankle. (Photo 4-1)

Lying on the floor like this, move your left hip around a little. How does it feel to move the hip? Is the motion clear to you? Does the hip move easily in all directions? Is the motion smooth or is it jerky in spots? Does it require a lot of effort to move the hip or does the motion feel easy? Take a few minutes and explore the motion of the hip

Now move the left hip forward very slowly in the direction in which you're looking. (Photo 4-2) Move the

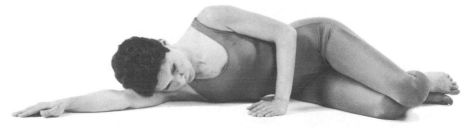

Photo 4-2: *Move your left hip forward a little so that your left knee moves out in front of your right knee.*

hip only as far as is easy and then return to your initial position. Repeat the motion, paying attention to all details. Notice how the left knee moves out in front of the right knee a little as the hip moves forward. Think about your right side, lying on the floor. Can you feel the weight shift on the floor as the hip moves? Can you feel the pressure change in the palm of the left hand? Make 25 repetitions of this hip motion and then stop.

Now move the left hip back, opposite the direction in which you were moving before. Move the hip back as far as is easy and then return to the initial position. (Photo 4-3) Again make 25 movements and then stop. As you move, notice how the left knee moves back behind the right knee and how the pressure of the right side against the floor changes.

Now move the left hip forward and back so that the left knee comes out in front of the right and then moves behind it. As you move the hip, reach up with the left hand and use the hand to feel the motion of the hip. (Photos 4-4, 4-5) Does the hand feel as if it's moving straight forward and back? Make another 25 repetitions and then turn onto your back and rest.

As you lie on your back, pay attention to your hips and how they rest on the floor. Compare the left hip with the right. Which hip feels bigger? Which feels higher off the floor?

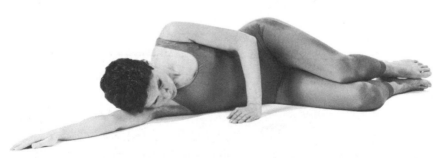

Photo 4-3: *Now move your left hip backward as far as is easy and then return to your initial position.*

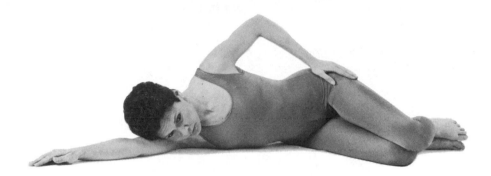

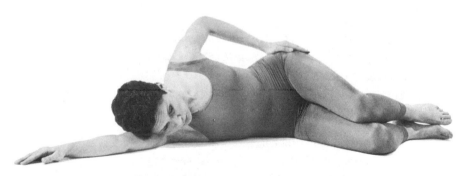

Photos 4-4, 4-5: *Now move your left hip forward and backward; use your hand to feel the motion of the hip as you do this.*

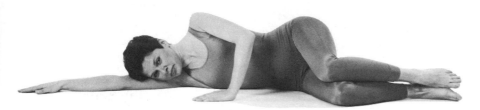

Photo 4-6: *Lie on your right side as before and move your hip up in the direction of your head.*

Turn and lie on your right side as before, with the legs drawn up, one on top of the other, the head resting on the right arm, and the palm of the left hand on the floor in front. Move the hip in the direction of the head a little and then let the hip move back to its resting position. (Photo 4-6) Continue to move like this and think about your waist in the area where you wear your belt. As the left hip moves up toward the head, can you feel that this area presses against the floor so that the gap between the floor and the body gets smaller? Make 25 motions of the hip and then stop.

Now reach over the top of the head with the left hand and place the palm of that hand on top of your head. The tips of the fingers will be close to or touching the right ear and the left elbow will point straight up toward the ceiling. (Photo 4-7) Move the hip up toward the head as before, but this time, as the hip moves up, also raise the head a little so that the left ear moves toward the left hip; use the left arm to help lift the head. (Photo 4-8) Repeat this move 25 times, stop, and replace the left hand on the floor in front of you. Now move the hip up toward the head a few times without lifting the head. How does the hip motion feel now? Is it larger? Easier?

Now move the hip down away from the head. (Photo 4-9) Move it down as far as is easy, then return to the initial position. Repeat the motion 25 times, noticing what happens in the rest of your body as the hip moves. Pay attention to your waist. Can you feel that this area rises up

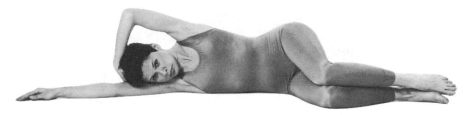

Photo 4-7: *Place your left hand on top of your head with fingertips near your right ear; your elbow points toward the ceiling.*

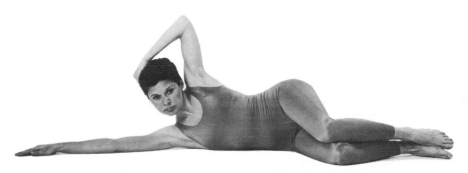

Photo 4-8: *Use your left hand to help lift your head and at the same time move your hip up toward your head.*

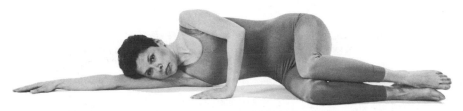

Photo 4-9: *Now move your hip away from your head so that you create a small space between your waist and the floor.*

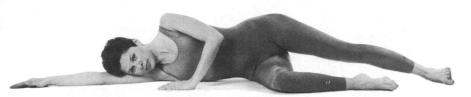

Photo 4-10: *Straighten your left leg out, heel resting on the floor, and flex your left ankle.*

and that the gap increases between the waist and the floor as the hip moves?

Now straighten your left leg, aligning it with your body, with the left heel resting on the floor. Flex your left foot so that the toes come closer to the left knee. (Photo 4-10) From this position slide the left heel down the floor away from your head and then let it come back up. (Photo 4-11) Repeat this move 25 times, then stop and replace the left leg on top of the right.

Now move the left hip up and down so that the hip approaches the head and then moves away from it. (Photos 4-12, 4-13) Repeat this motion 25 times. As you do this, let your attention move around your body. Notice how the pressure shifts on the right hip and how the area near where you wear your belt moves up and down on the floor. Think about the ribs on the right side. What can you

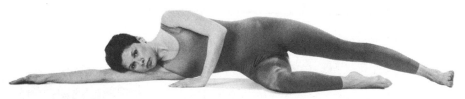

Photo 4-11: *Keeping your left knee straight, slide your left heel away from your head, creating a small gap between your waist and the floor.*

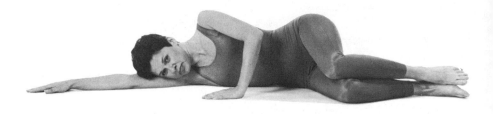

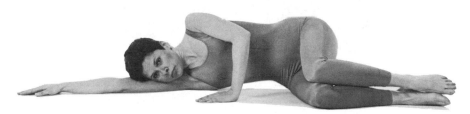

Photos 4-12, 4-13: *Now move your left hip up and down so that your hip approaches your head and then moves away.*

feel there? Notice your head. Does the head move around on the right arm as the left hip moves? Continue to move the hip and place your left hand on your hip. Does the hand feel as if it is moving straight up and down, closer to the head and farther away from it? After 25 repetitions, turn and lie on your back and rest.

As you lie there, compare the feeling in the left and right hips. Which hip feels bigger? Which hip feels closer to the head? Think about the left and right legs. Which one feels longer?

Again turn and lie on your right side with your legs drawn up and your head resting comfortably on your right arm. Move the left hip up and down a few times and then forward and back. Notice how the up-and-down motion draws a straight line, and how the forward-and-backward motion also draws a straight line, at right angles to the first line. Explore these two motions for a few minutes. Are the two "lines" really at right angles? Are the four arms of the cross figure formed by the two lines of equal length?

Now imagine that the center of the cross is the center of a circle and slowly draw that circle with the left hip. It doesn't have to be a big circle—even a radius of an inch or two will do. As you move, pay careful attention to the motion of the hip. Is it a true circle or are there flat spots or places where the motion is jerky or stiff? Draw about 10 or 15 circles in one direction and then reverse and draw another 10 or 15 circles in the opposite direction. Use your left hand to check the circles in the same way that you used it to check the up-and-down and forward-and-back motions of the hip. (Photo 4-14) A circle contains all directions, so if you can easily move your hip in a circle, then the hip will be free to move properly when you run.

As you make the circles, let your attention wander around to the rest of your body. Because you are moving the pelvis—the largest bone in the body, with many strong connections to the other parts of the body—you should be able to feel some motion wherever you direct your attention. Can you feel your weight shift on the floor? What does your head do as the hip moves in a circle? Notice your breathing. Is it smooth and easy as you draw

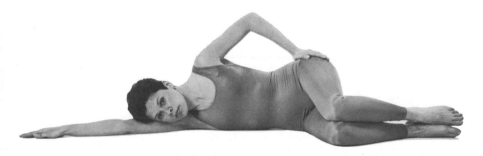

Photo 4-14: *Move your left hip in a circle; use your left hand to feel the circular motion you are making.*

the circles? Stop making the circles and just move your hip around however you wish, as you did when you first lay down on the floor. How does the motion of the hip feel now? Lie on your back and rest.

As you lie there, roll one leg left and right on the floor so that the toes move left and right, pivoting about the heel, which remains where it is on the floor. Roll one leg a few times and then roll the other. Compare the efforts required to roll the two legs. Which is easier?

Very slowly roll over to one side, come up onto your hands and knees, and stand up. Notice how it feels to stand after working one side of the body like this. Do you feel a little lopsided? Walk around a little and try swinging the hips and shoulders. Which hip moves more easily? Lie down and rest.

Slowly turn and lie on your left side. Stretch your left arm out on the floor overhead and rest your left ear on your arm. Draw up your legs so that the knees and hips are bent at right angles and place the palm of the right hand on the floor in front of your chest.

Go through the motions with the right hip that you just made with the left hip, but this time do the motions *mentally*. Don't actually move anything. Begin by "moving" the right hip forward. Go just far enough to detect the increase in tension in the muscles around the hip, as if the hip were just getting ready to move, and then cease all effort. Repeat each "movement" only five times and stop.

"Move" the right hip forward five times, then backward, and then forward and backward. Then, "move" the right hip up and down, remembering to "lift" the head with the right hand, straighten the right leg on the floor, and "move" it up and down the floor. Finally, draw circles in both directions. Pay attention to your breathing as you do these imaginary movements. Be sure to lie on your back and check the results after each set of "movements."

When you are finished with the right hip, lie on your back and compare the feeling in the left and right hips. Roll one leg left and right, then the other. Now which leg rolls more easily?

Slowly roll onto one side and stand up. Walk around a

little using your normal walk and then try swinging your hips and shoulders in the exaggerated way that we have been using. How do your hips feel?

Think about the movements that you just did. With the left hip, you repeated each motion 25 times and the whole series probably took about 30 minutes to complete. With the right hip, you only *imagined* the motions and repeated each one only 5 times. Nevertheless, you will almost certainly feel that the improvement in the right hip is as much or even more than the improvement in the left.

There is a lesson about exercising in this paradox: If we can get equal or greater improvement by just imagining a motion, why should we spend our time on endless repetitions of a particular move? If you repeat the same move, such as running, over and over again in the same way, you will just be practicing your old, imperfect way of running. Consequently, you'll just become more and more entrenched in the particular way that you run. And if that way of running is out of balance, you will ultimately damage your body. This kind of training will build your stamina, of course, but it will also cause you more pain.

But this doesn't have to be the case. By gently exploring the motions of the body in a slow, nonstressful way as you have just done, you can change for the better the *way* that you run by reducing the stress and effort required. This will also increase your stamina, but in a roundabout way: As your running becomes more efficient you will need less energy to run, which means you'll be able to go farther on a given amount of energy. Remember Bif? That's what happened to him, until he eventually outran his poor dog.

Naomi: The "John Wayne" Approach

Once when I was teaching a weekend workshop, Carla, one of the participants, asked me if I would evaluate Naomi, her 13-year-old daughter.

"What would you like me to do for her?" I asked.

Carla launched into a long story. The problem, she said, was that Naomi's feet turned out to the side when she walked instead of pointing straight ahead. Someone at school, a PE instructor probably, had pointed this out and warned that it would cause problems for Naomi unless she started walking correctly. So Naomi had tried to walk with her feet straight forward. This worked fine— as long as she was thinking about it. As soon as her attention was distracted, however, her feet fell back into their old habits. After a week Naomi got bored with the whole thing and refused to "walk right," in spite of dire predictions from everyone that she would get flat feet, have lower back problems, and suffer numerous other ailments.

Various experts had been consulted and they all agreed that Naomi's walk needed improvement. But no one could come up with a concrete method for improving it.

"Does she have any pain or disability?" I asked.

"No," said Carla.

"How about sports? Does she participate in any sports at all?"

"Naomi plays softball and she's pretty good," Carla replied.

"Well," I said, "maybe there isn't really a problem. If there's no pain, and she moves well enough to play ball, it may just be that that's the way she moves. Sometimes you find people who move differently from the average, just like you find people who are considerably shorter or taller than the average. It's not wrong, it's just different."

"Still," said Carla, "I wish you could just look at her."

"When can you bring her in?" I asked.

"How about tomorrow at lunch?"

The next day at noon, Carla appeared with Naomi in tow. I asked Naomi to walk around for a while. Sure enough, her feet turned way out to the side as she walked. Not only that, but they were far apart from each other when they came down on the floor. I could see that Naomi was not doing much with her upper body as she walked and that this was causing the problems with her feet.

"Your mother tells me that you play softball. How do you like it?" I asked Naomi.

"It's my favorite," she said. "I play every day."

"What part of the game do you like best?" I asked.

"Throwing and hitting," she replied.

"How about running the bases? How do you like that?"

Naomi looked down at her feet. "That part's not as much fun."

It looked like Naomi did have a problem after all. Running with her feet turned out like that would probably be a big effort, and I would have bet that she wasn't very fast.

"Do you think you can do something for her?" her mother asked.

"Let me think about it for a minute," I said.

I tried to think of something I could do for Naomi in the little bit of time I had. I considered explaining to her that the position of the feet when they hit the ground during running is determined by how well the hips move; and that when the pelvis turns to take a step, the hip joint should move so that the thigh rotates opposite the pelvis, which allows the leg to move straight forward without rotating. And that for all of this to happen as it should, the shoulders must be moving correctly with respect to the hips. But that didn't seem like the right approach for a 13-year-old girl. So I decided to try something different.

"Do you know how John Wayne walks?" I asked Naomi.

"Sure," she said, "he walks like you wouldn't want to get in his way."

"Can you walk like that?" I asked.

Naomi jumped up from her chair and pulled herself up to her full height of 4 feet 11 inches. She cocked her head, fixed her eyes straight ahead in a good imitation of a steely glint, and clenched both fists. Then she began to stride across the floor with an exaggerated walking motion.

"Look at your feet," I said.

Naomi looked down at her feet. "They're *straight*," she said, half in disbelief.

I was feeling pretty cocky. My idea had worked even better than I had expected. "I've got another minute," I said to Carla. "Anything else you want fixed?"

"Wait a minute. Just what exactly did you do?" Carla asked.

"Well," I said, "the problem was that she wasn't swinging her hips and shoulders when she walked. When she did her 'John Wayne' walk she started swinging her hips and shoulders, and that made her feet come down in the right place.

"The problem wasn't in her feet at all, but in her upper body—her hips and shoulders. Everybody kept talking about feet, so Naomi was looking in the wrong place.

"When I teach that to adults, it usually takes a lot longer," I continued. "But with kids the movement patterns are much easier to change; sometimes they can pick up the idea in just a few seconds."

I looked at Naomi. "Try that again and notice what you do with your hips and shoulders to make it work." Naomi began to stride around the room again. "I'm just swinging them around, that's all," she said.

"Well, just remember how that feels and you won't have any more problems with your feet. Oh, and by the way, when you run the bases in softball, remember to do that same thing, but even more."

I turned back to Carla. "I really think that's going to do it," I said. "I don't see any big problems with her movement. Somehow, she just missed that little piece of learning, that's all. Now that she has that, I think she'll be fine."

5

The
Shoulders
Alone

In the previous chapter we worked with the hips, which
are the powerhouse of the body. For the power of the hips
to be effective in running, however, the motion of the hips
must be counterbalanced by the motion of the shoulders.
This is a crucial point and only now is it becoming understood in such a way that runners can use it to improve
their running.

Because of the human body's upright stance, the
power of the hips has to be directed all the way down our
long legs to the ground for it to be useful. However, when
we push at an angle at the end of a long lever, such as the
leg, we have to have some kind of opposing force or we
will get pushed off to one side and lose our balance.

Here's a way to feel how the power of the hips can be
wasted if it is not counterbalanced. Stand up and hold
your right leg straight out in front. Keep the knee straight
and the leg more or less parallel to the floor.

Have a friend grab your right foot and push it to your
right. (Photo 5-1) Holding the position that you are in,
try to resist the turning motion. You will find that, even if

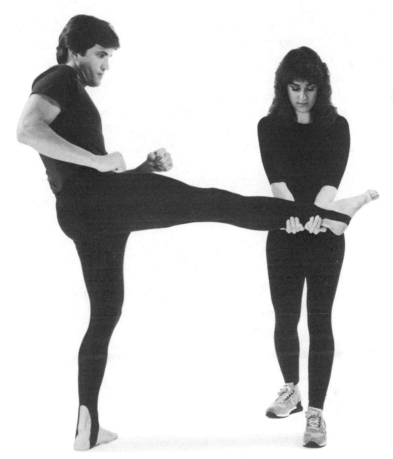

Photo 5-1: *With your leg straight out in front of you, have a friend push your leg to the side; try to resist*

you are unusually large and strong and your friend is not, it is impossible to resist the turning motion. In this position, you have nothing to push against and your strength is useless.

If you try this same experiment while holding on to something solid, such as the bannister of some stairs, you will find that it's a different story. Now that you have something to push against, your friend will have a much more difficult time pushing your foot off to the side.

Providing this kind of support is exactly the function

of the shoulders and arms during running. The motion of the shoulders and arms gives the hips and legs something to "push against" as they move.

To begin working with the shoulders, lie down on your right side. Draw your knees up along the floor so that both the knee joints and hip joints are bent at approximate right angles. The legs should be together, so that the left knee lies over the right knee and the left foot lies over the right foot. Stretch the right arm out comfortably on the floor overhead and rest your right ear

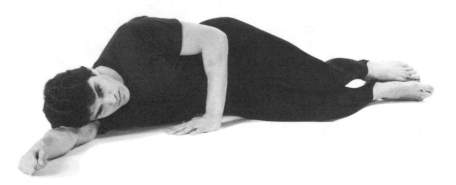

Photo 5-2: *Lie on your right side and bend your knees and hips at right angles; rest your head on your right arm and place your left hand on the floor in front of your chest.*

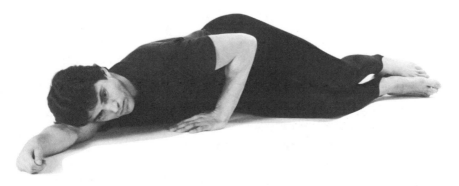

Photo 5-3: *Move your left shoulder straight forward a little in the direction in which you are looking.*

on it. Place the palm of the left hand on the floor just in front of your chest, with the elbow and shoulder joints bent at right angles. (Photo 5-2)

In this position, slowly move the left shoulder around a little. Does the shoulder move easily in all directions, or more easily in some directions than in others? Is the whole movement smooth or are there some areas where the shoulder moves easily and others where the motion feels stiff or jerky?

Now move the shoulder straight forward, in the direction in which you are looking, and then let it come back to the neutral position. (Photo 5-3) Repeat this move slowly, about 25 times. As you move, pay attention to the quality of the motion; don't try to move as far or as fast as you can. Move the shoulder forward just far enough so that you can get a clear feel for the motion and then let the shoulder move easily back to its initial position.

Now move the left shoulder back in the opposite direction. (Photo 5-4) Move it slowly, just as far as you can without straining, and then let it come back to a resting position. Repeat the motion about 20 times. As you move, pay careful attention to the direction of the shoulder's motion. Is the motion really straight backward or does the shoulder move up toward the head or down toward the feet a little? Is the motion a straight line or does it curve?

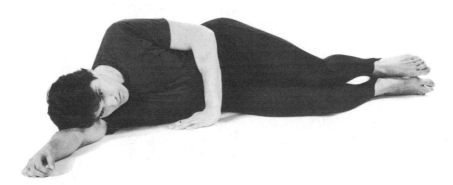

Photo 5-4: *Now move your left shoulder back in the opposite direction; move it as far as you can without straining.*

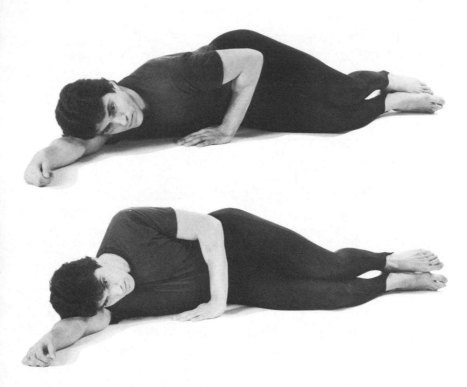

Photos 5-5, 5-6: *Continue to move your shoulder forward and backward, passing the midpoint without stopping.*

In order to notice all these small details of motion, you must move slowly and easily and pay careful attention to what you're doing.

Continue to move the shoulder forward and backward, passing through the middle point without stopping. (Photos 5-5, 5-6) Again, notice all the details of the motion. Does the shoulder move forward as far as it moves backward? Is the whole motion a straight line? Repeat the motion about 25 times and then lie on your back and rest.

As you lie there, notice your left and right shoulders. Compare the way the two shoulders lie against the floor. Which shoulder is higher up off the floor? Take a few minutes to lie still and just appreciate the difference between the two shoulders.

Now turn and lie on your right side, with your head resting on your right arm and your knees and hips at right angles, as before. Rest the palm of your left hand on the floor just in front of your chest.

Move your left shoulder straight up toward your left ear and then let the shoulder come back to the initial position. (Photo 5-7) Repeat the motion, moving slowly, about 25 times. Again, pay attention to all the details of the motion. Does the shoulder move straight up toward the ear, or does it move toward the front or the back a little?

Now move the left shoulder down, away from the left ear. (Photo 5-8) Again repeat the motion about 25 times.

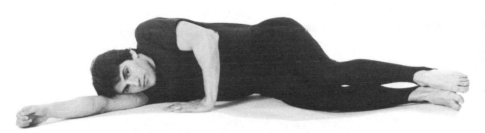

Photo 5-7: *Move your shoulder straight up toward your left ear and then let it come back to a resting position.*

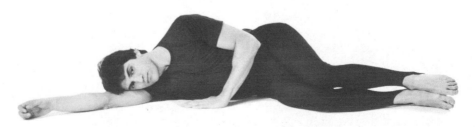

Photo 5-8: *Move your shoulder down away from your head a little and then back to its resting position.*

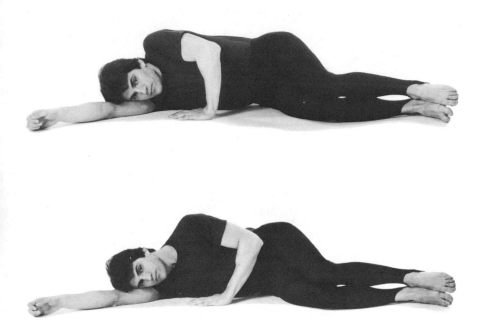

Photos 5-9, 5-10: *Move your shoulder up and down, toward your left ear and away from it, without stopping midway.*

Rest briefly and then move the shoulder up and down, toward the left ear and then away from it, without stopping in the middle. (Photos 5-9, 5-10) Is the motion a straight line or is it curved? Does the shoulder move smoothly or are there rough spots in the motion? Repeat this motion about 25 times, stop, lie on your back, and rest.

As you lie there, compare the feeling in the left and right shoulders. Mentally measure the distance between the left ear and left shoulder and between the right ear and right shoulder. Are the two distances equal? Take a minute or two to lie still and evaluate the differences between the two shoulders.

Turn and lie on your right side as before, with the legs drawn up and your head resting on the right arm. Think about the series of movements you've made with the left shoulder until now. First you moved the shoulder forward, then back, and then forward and back. Move the shoulder forward and back like this a few times and notice that the shoulder draws a straight line in the air as it moves.

The second series of moves involved moving the shoulder up, then down, and then up and down. Move the shoulder up and down a few times and notice that the shoulder again draws a straight line, at right angles to the first line.

Spend a few minutes exploring these two moves and notice that the two lines make a cross in the air. When you can get a clear picture of this cross, imagine that the center of the cross is the center of a circle, and with the shoulder draw a circle in the air, centered on the cross. (Photo 5-11) Make about 20 clockwise circles and then about 20 counterclockwise circles. Does the motion feel like a true circle or are there flat spots? Lie on your back and rest. As you lie there, think of the two shoulders. Notice how each shoulder makes contact with the floor and how far each shoulder is from the head.

Again turn and lie on the right side, legs drawn up as before and head resting on the right arm. With the left hand, reach over the top of the head. Place the palm of

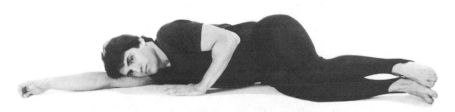

Photo 5-11: *Move your left shoulder in a circle; does the motion feel like a true circle or are there jerky spots?*

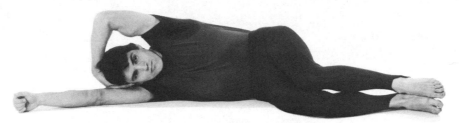

Photo 5-12: *Place your left hand on top of your head, fingertips near the right ear and elbow pointing upward.*

the left hand on top of the head so that the fingers just touch the right ear. The left elbow should be pointing up toward the ceiling. (Photo 5-12)

Use the left hand to help lift the head up a little. Lift the head slowly and notice how the left elbow moves toward the left hip just a bit; then let the head back down until it rests on the right arm. (Photo 5-13) As you move, pay attention to the spine in back. Where does the spine bend to lift the head? Notice your ribs on the left side. Do the ribs move at all when you lift the head? Repeat this move about 15 times and then rest, lying on your side, with the left hand on the floor in front of you.

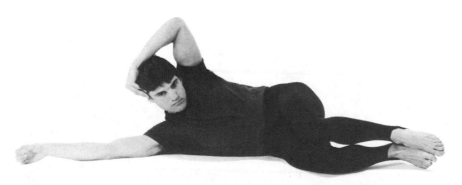

Photo 5-13: *Using your left hand to help, lift your head up slowly, then let it back down to rest on your right arm.*

Once again, draw some circles with your shoulder while lying on your side. How do the circles feel now? Are they easier to draw? Smoother? Lie on your back and rest, and as you lie there notice the breathing motion in the upper chest on the left and right sides. Which side of your chest feels bigger? Which side seems to be taking in more air?

After a minute or so, slowly turn onto one side and get up onto your feet. Notice how your two shoulders feel. Go and look in a mirror and compare your left and right shoulders. Which shoulder looks broader?

Walk around a little and try swinging your hips and shoulders in the manner suggested in Chapter 1. Notice the big difference bctween the two shoulders. Which shoulder moves more easily?

Lie down on your back. Turn onto your left side, draw up your knees, and rest your head on your left arm. Mentally review the moves that you just went through with the left shoulder. First you drew a cross, beginning with the forward and then the backward direction, and then you drew the up-and-down directions. Then you did circles in two directions, then you lifted the head with the left arm.

Go through this whole series of moves again, but moving the right shoulder. Is the right shoulder easier or more difficult to move than the left?

After you complete the motions on the right side, stand up and walk around. Again try swinging your shoulders and hips in the exaggerated way suggested in the first chapter. How does the shoulder motion feel now? How much do you think this will improve your running?

Rob: Movement and the Mind

After a class one evening, Rob, one of my students, stopped me on the way out to my car.

"Have you got a few minutes? I want to ask you about something," he said.

"Sure," I said, "what is it?"

"Well, I had a really strange experience while running the other day," he began, "and I think it's connected to the class. It's really got me baffled.

"I was doing some light running, and I was thinking about my shoulders and hips, and sort of mulling over some of the things you had talked about in class. I had only gone about a half-mile, and all of a sudden I felt something kind of slip down near my pelvis, and then— this is the really strange part—I had the distinct feeling that I was falling over backward."

"Did you actually fall?" I asked.

"No, that was what was so strange. I really felt as if I were falling, but I didn't fall. What do you make of that?"

"I'm pretty sure that I know what happened to you," I said, "but first, tell me what happened just after you felt that you were falling."

"Well, the whole thing really caught me by surprise and I stopped running. I felt kind of disoriented for a few seconds, and then that passed. I couldn't figure out what had happened, so I just started to run again."

"That's it? Nothing more?"

"Well," Rob said, "there was one other thing, but I didn't mention it because it doesn't make any sense. When I started running again, I felt like I was taller somehow."

"That makes a lot of sense," I said, "and it makes it easier for me to answer your question. What happened was you stopped compressing your body while you run."

Rob gave me a blank look. "I don't know what you're talking about."

"That compression, which is something that almost everyone does to some extent, consists of pulling your head down into your chest and actually shortening your entire body, particularly your spine," I explained. "Most people, when they think they're going to make some kind of effort, such as running, stiffen the body by contracting the muscles of the trunk. This has the effect of pulling the head down. It also constricts the breathing and ties up that motion of the hips and shoulders that I am always talking about."

"I still don't follow you," Rob said. "And what's all that got to do with the feeling of falling over backward?"

"That's the toughest part to explain because the subjective feeling is so strong, and yet it's caused by what looks like a very small change in posture.

"Everyone has a posture that is as unique as his voice and, like the voice, it's usually not as good as it could be. If you really change your running, you will change your posture, too. That's what happened to you. With most people the change is slow and they're not really aware of it. With you it was very abrupt, and you actually felt as if you were going to fall."

"How do you know this?" asked Rob. "I've never heard or read of anything like that anywhere."

"I'll bet you've never taken a running course like this before, either," I said.

"That's true," Rob admitted.

"Well, I'll tell you. When I was developing the ideas that I teach in this course, the same thing happened to me. In fact, it happened several times. One of those times was particularly powerful, and just after it happened I observed that the shape of my neck had changed. It took me some time to figure out that I was carrying my head in a very different way and that, in fact, my whole posture had changed."

"So what you're saying is that I stopped compressing my body as a result of the exercises that we did in the course, is that right?" Rob asked.

"That's right."

"That sounds pretty strange, but at least it explains how I could feel taller. But I still don't see how I could feel like I was falling backward like I did. In fact, the more I think about that, the stranger it seems."

"You're getting me into a corner now," I told Rob, "because it's hard to explain a subjective experience. But I know what you mean when you say it's strange. When it happened to me, I couldn't think of anything else for days afterward.

"But think about this. The entire nervous output of the brain consists solely of nerve impulses directed to muscles. In other words, all the nerve impulses that come out of the brain are devoted to producing movement. What you can deduce from that is that a lot—maybe most—of what goes on in the brain is devoted to controlling movement. If you change your posture in that way, you are changing the activity of a lot of the nerve cells in the brain. When that happens quickly, as it did to you, it can be pretty disorienting."

"Well, I don't know," Rob said. "Those are really different ideas. I want to think about them for a while. Maybe you're right. I guess the important thing is that I'm really running better, and that's why I came to the class."

6

Hips and Shoulders Together

In the previous two chapters we worked to improve awareness of each hip and each shoulder as individual units. Now we'll explore moving the hips and shoulders together.

When running, especially on broken terrain, you need to be able to move the hips and shoulders in a number of different ways relative to each other. And if you participate in a sport such as soccer or football, you have to be able to run in such a way that you can turn and pivot rapidly, on a moment's notice. To do this without losing balance, the shoulders and hips must be free to move in any direction so that they can counterbalance each other as you turn, accelerate, and stop.

To begin exploring the motions of the hips and shoulders, lie down on your right side, draw up your knees, and rest your head on your right arm. Bend your knees and hips at right angles. The left knee and foot

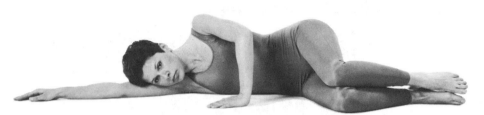

Photo 6-1: *Lie on your right side and draw up your knees so that your knees and hips are bent at right angles.*

should be on top of the right knee and foot. Place the palm of the left hand on the floor just in front of the chest so that the left elbow is bent at a right angle and the forearm is approximately vertical. (Photo 6-1)

Move the left hip and shoulder forward and backward together. (Photos 6-2, 6-3) Continue this motion and let your attention move through your body. Notice how your right side rolls forward and back along the floor and how your head rolls along the right arm. Think about the left knee and elbow. The knee and elbow should go forward and back together. Let the left hip and shoulder move forward and back like this about 25 times, in an easy, effortless motion, and then stop.

Now stretch the left arm out straight, in line with the torso, so that the hand rests on the floor overhead. Then stretch the left leg out straight on the floor, in line with the torso, so that the left foot rests on the floor. The left arm and leg are in a straight line with the body. (Photo 6-4) Holding this position, swing the entire left side of the body forward and back so that the chest comes closer to the

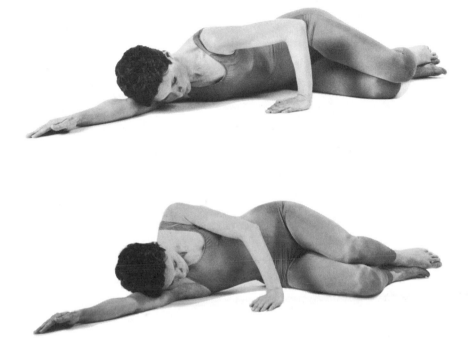

Photos 6-2, 6-3: *Move your left hip and shoulder forward and backward together.*

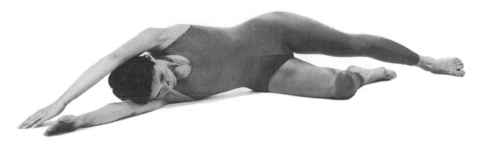

Photo 6-4: *Straighten your left arm and leg out so that your left hand and foot rest on the floor.*

floor in front and then moves away from it. (Photos 6-5, 6-6) Continue to move like this and notice that the left shoulder and hip are still moving forward and back. Repeat this move about 25 times; then bring your left leg back on top of your right, replace the palm of your left hand on the floor in front of your chest, and rest for a minute, lying on your side.

Now move the left hip forward and the left shoulder backward, then reverse the motion, moving the left hip

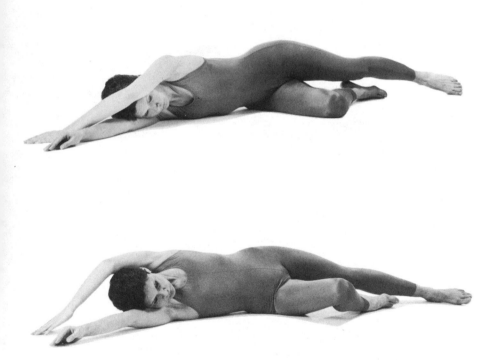

Photos 6-5, 6-6: *Swing the entire left side of your body forward and backward so that your chest comes closer to the floor and then moves away from it.*

backward and the left shoulder forward. Continue like
this with the left hip and shoulder moving in opposite
directions. (Photos 6-7, 6-8) Notice how your right side
rolls against the floor. Does the motion of the right side
follow the left hip or the left shoulder? Think of your
breathing as you move. Is your breathing slow and easy or
do you hold your breath at certain points in the motion?
Repeat the motion about 25 times or more. Stop, roll onto
your back, and rest.

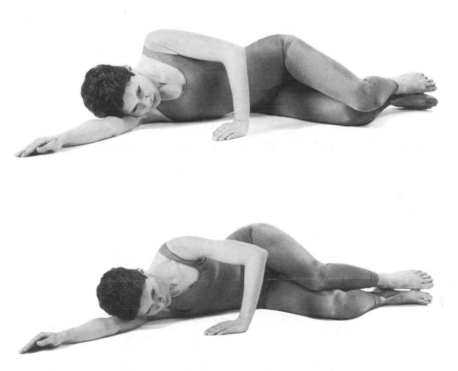

Photos 6-7, 6-8: *Now move your left hip forward and your
left shoulder backward, then reverse the motion, moving the
left hip backward and the left shoulder forward.*

   As you lie there, compare the feelings in the left and right sides of your body. Mentally measure the distance between the left hip and shoulder and the right hip and shoulder. Which is greater? How is the breathing in the left and right ribs? Can you feel any difference between the left eye and the right eye? Take a few minutes to assess the changes that have occurred in your body.

   Turn and lie on your right side as before, with the knees drawn up and the head resting on the right arm. Move your left shoulder and hip up and down together, closer to the head and then farther away from it. (Photos 6-9, 6-10) Notice how the entire left side of the body

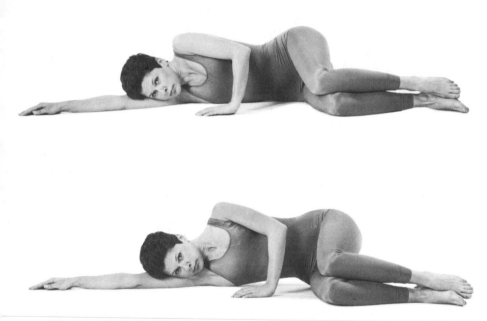

Photos 6-9, 6-10: *Move your shoulder and hip up and down together, closer to your head and then farther away. As you move your hip down, you should create a small space between your waist and the floor.*

moves up and down. Can you feel that the area just above your hip, on the right side, moves closer to the floor and then away from it as the right hip rolls on the floor? Repeat this motion about 25 times, then stop and rest, lying on your side.

Next move the left hip down away from the head and the left shoulder up toward the head. As you do this, the hip and shoulder will move farther away from each other. Then reverse this motion and move the shoulder down and the hip up; in this movement, the shoulder and hip approach each other. (Photos 6-11, 6-12) Continue like this, moving the left shoulder and hip farther away from

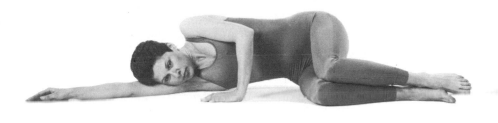

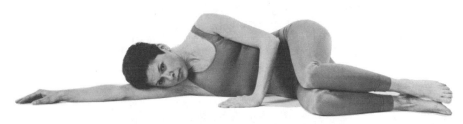

Photos 6-11, 6-12: *Move your left hip down away from your head and your left shoulder up toward your head. Then reverse this motion and move your shoulder down and your hip up.*

each other and then closer to each other. Notice how the ribs on the left side contract a little as the shoulder and hip approach each other and then expand as the shoulder and hip move away from each other. Repeat this move about 25 times and then stop and rest, lying on your side.

Stretch your left arm out straight, in line with the torso, so that the hand rests on the floor overhead. Then stretch your left leg out straight on the floor, in line with the torso and the left arm, so that the left foot rests on the floor. Flex the left foot, bringing the toes toward the knees.

From this position, slide the left hand down the floor closer to the head and at the same time slide the left heel up the floor closer to the head. The left hand and foot will move closer to each other. Then reverse the motion, sliding the left hand straight up on the floor away from the head and the left heel down the floor away from the head. The left hand and foot will now move farther away from each other. Continue this motion, moving the left hand

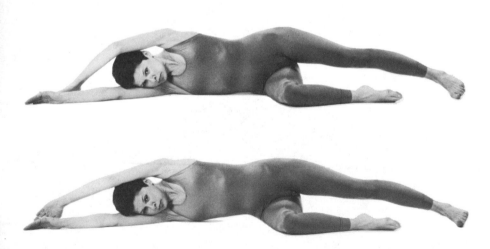

Photos 6-13, 6-14: *With left arm and leg stretched out on the floor, move your left hand and foot closer together; then reverse the motion and move them away from each other.*

and foot closer to each other and then farther away. Make sure that the left knee and elbow remain straight. (Photos 6-13, 6-14) The hand and foot will only move a short distance, just a few inches.

As you do this, pay attention to what is going on in the center of your body. Notice how the ribs on the left side are compressed as the hand and foot come closer to each other and then open up as the hand and foot move away from each other. Repeat this move about 25 times, moving slowly and breathing easily, and then turn onto your back and rest.

As you lie there, compare the feeling in the left and right sides of your body. Notice the breathing motion in the left and right ribs, and which side lies flatter against the floor. Which leg feels longer, the left or the right? Take a minute or two to fully appreciate all the differences between the two sides.

Turn and lie again on your right side, with the knees drawn up and the head resting comfortably on the right arm. With the left hand, reach over the top of the head and grasp the head with the hand. The palm of the hand rests on top of the head and the fingers of the hand should be close to or actually touching the right ear. (Photo 6-15)

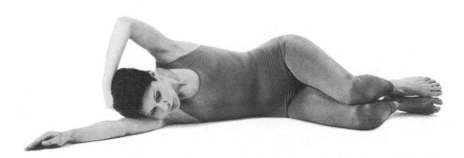

Photo 6-15: *Place your left hand on top of your head, fingertips near the right ear and elbow pointing upward.*

From this position, lift your head up to the side so that the left ear moves toward the left hip. Use the left hand to help lift the head. Lift the head just a little bit and then set it back down. Repeat this move slowly and notice how the left hip moves toward the head as the head and left hand raise up. (Photo 6-16) Raise and lower the head about 10 times and then raise the head up and stop.

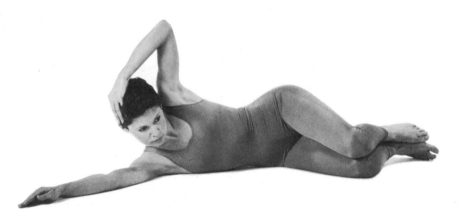

Photo 6-16: *Using your left hand to help, lift your head just a little and then set it back down.*

With the head up and the left hand still on the head, roll the whole left side of the body forward and back a little, making sure that you don't hold your breath. (Photos 6-17, 6-18) Roll about 10 or 15 times, lower the head back down to rest on the right arm, and set the palm of the left hand on the floor in front.

As you lie there, move the left hip and shoulder around a little. How does the motion feel? Are both parts of the motion smooth and easy? Turn and lie on the left side and move the right hip and shoulder around, comparing the motion of the right side to that of the left side. Which side moves more easily? Turn and lie on your back and rest for a minute.

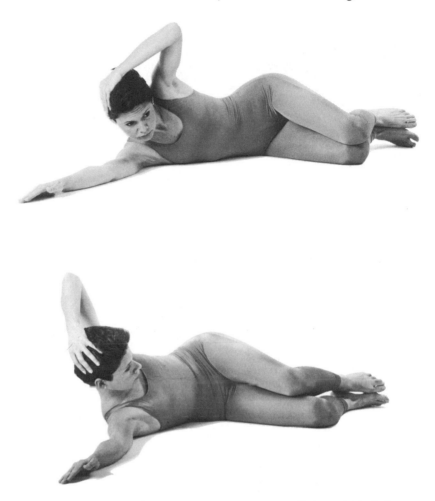

Photos 6-17, 6-18: *With your head up, roll the whole left side of your body forward and backward a little, making sure that you don't hold your breath.*

Now turn and lie on the right side. Move the left hip and shoulder up toward the head and stop. Then move the hip and shoulder forward, then down, then back, and then up, drawing a circle with the hip and shoulder at the same time. (Photo 6-19) Draw about 20 circles one way and then another 20 moving in the opposite direction. Pay

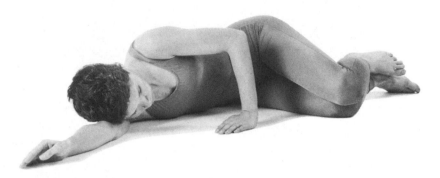

Photo 6-19: *Now move your left hip and shoulder in circles together; move both in as true a circle as possible.*

careful attention to the movements of the hip and shoulder, making sure that each moves in a true circle. Stop and rest on your side.

Now move the left hip back and the left shoulder forward, and then stop. From this position, move the shoulder down and the hip up, just a little, in an arc. Just begin to draw the two circles, then reverse the motion and go back to the starting point. Move the hip and shoulder again, and this time go a little farther. Continue like this until you can draw these two circles at the same time.

You may find that you can't do this move right away. Moving the hip and shoulder in circles in the same direction but starting at different points on the circles is a fairly tricky move. Spend a few minutes at this and then let it go. Give this exercise a few days to sink into your body, then try it again. You will be surprised at how much easier it is.

Turn and lie on your back, rest for a minute, and then stand up. Compare the left and right sides of your body. Walk around a little and swing the hips and shoulders. Which side moves more easily?

After a few minutes of this, lie down on your left side, draw up your knees, and rest your head on your left arm. Go back through the same series of moves with the right hip and shoulder, and improve that side also.

After you have done both sides, stand up and walk around. As you walk, think about the hip and shoulder circles that you just made. Try to use this motion as you walk, allowing your hips and shoulders to "roll" as you walk along. While walking, don't try to make exact circles, but just let the hips and shoulders move in an easy, more or less circular motion. Walk a little way and then gradually speed up into a slow jogging motion, still rolling your hips and shoulders. Notice the smooth, coordinated feeling that this motion gives to your running.

Susan: Does Running Have to Be Painful?

After the last session of one of my running classes, everyone was in a fine mood and most of us went out to dinner at a local restaurant.

The conversation at dinner centered on movement and ways to improve it. Many people talked about pain and whether it was necessary to endure a lot of pain to learn to run well, or to learn to play tennis, or to ski.

As the conversation progressed, a few people remarked that during the class a lot of their chronic aches and pains had diminished or disappeared entirely. This started the group thinking, and pretty soon almost everyone admitted to having had some kind of ache or pain that had gone away during the course of the class.

Finally, a woman named Susan summed up the group mood. "We all took the class to learn to run a little better," said Susan, "and besides learning to run differently, we have managed to get rid of all kinds of painful knees, aching backs, and stiff necks. How can learning to run in a slightly different way do all that?"

Everyone looked at me expectantly. "If you remember," I began, "at the beginning of the first class I mentioned that most of what we were going to do in the class was taken from the work of a man named Moshe Feldenkrais. Feldenkrais himself started out with a bad knee. Around 1925, when he was 22 years old and living in France, one of his knees was practically destroyed in a soccer match. The knee was bent at almost a right angle straight out to the side, and most of the internal and external ligaments were strained or torn.

"At that time, surgical techniques for repairing damaged knees were nowhere near as advanced as they are now, and so Feldenkrais had a pretty rough time of it. In fact, he managed to damage his other knee while walking around favoring the bad one. But through perseverance and lots of study, Feldenkrais found a way to rehabilitate and use his knee again, and he developed the ideas that were to become the foundation of his method of movement.

"What Feldenkrais had discovered was that by working with movement you can improve the organization of the entire nervous system in a way that has not been well understood until recently. Getting rid of aches and pains is kind of a side effect or fringe benefit of learning to use your nervous system in a more harmonious way—which is the basis of the Feldenkrais Method. Many people explore the Feldenkrais Method to get rid of chronic pain, and so the method is becoming well known as a means for relieving pain, but there is a lot more to it than that.

"One of the things I'm trying to do with this running class is to show how Feldenkrais's ideas about learning can be applied in a direct way to produce incredible improvements in performance in a very short period of time. Most of you have experienced lots of improvement during our classes, but even those improvements barely scratch the surface of the Feldenkrais Method. His method is a basic discovery about human functioning that is comparable in importance with basic discoveries about the physical world that were made in the last century and the early part of this one by men like Maxwell, Einstein, Planck, and Bohr.

"Anyway—have I answered your question, Susan?"

"Well, not quite," she said. "You said that this 'better

organization' gets rid of pains. Could you give a specific example of how that works?"

"Sure, how about this: Have you ever heard that most people carry more weight on one leg than the other? Well, if you run a lot, and use one leg more than the other, that leg can become painful, because it's doing more than its share of the work.

"In order to balance out the two legs, though, you have to balance the muscles in the hips and all along the spine and up into the neck also. You can't just shift your weight a little onto the other leg. That only works as long as you are thinking about it.

"This balancing out of the two sides of the body so that they move in a more symmetrical way is part of what I mean when I talk about better organization. And when this balancing takes place, your aches and pains will disappear, too."

"Well, that makes plenty of sense," said Susan. "Thanks for taking the time to explain it."

7

Hips and Shoulders Standing

When we run, especially on broken terrain, we have to be able to move our hips, shoulders, and legs in a variety of ways. While the hips are rotating to the left and right, the hip, knee, and ankle joints must be able to flex and extend to deal with the ups and downs of the terrain.

To do this efficiently we should be able to flex and extend the three joints in the leg while moving the hips and shoulders in a variety of different ways. Here is a way to test your ability to move in this way—and to improve it.

First we'll explore the turning motion of the body with the hips and shoulders moving in the same direction. Next we'll spend a few minutes bending the joints of the legs, and then we'll combine these two motions in several different ways. After that we'll turn the hips and shoulders in opposite directions, as we do when we walk or run, and again we will bend the knees. Finally we will see that this leads to a particular kind of movement involving the hips, shoulders, and legs that is very valuable as a coordination exercise for runners.

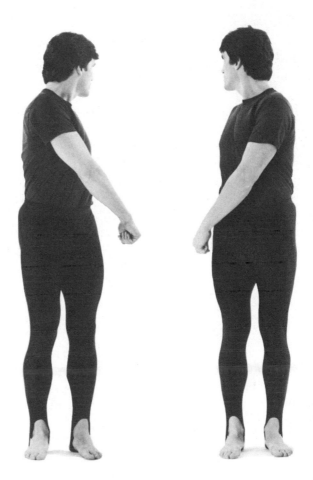

Photos 7-1, 7-2: *Stand up and turn your whole body—hips, shoulders, head, and eyes—to the left and right.*

Stand up and turn your whole body to the left and back to the right in an easy, twisting motion. (Photos 7-1, 7-2) Continue to turn like this, looking to the left as you turn left and to the right as you turn right.

Move your attention down to your feet. Notice how your weight shifts to the left side of your feet as you turn to the left and then to the right side as you turn back to the right.

Let your attention move up to your ankles and notice how the ankle joints move. Notice how the lower legs rotate to the left and then back to the right as you turn.

Move your attention from your legs to your hips. Notice how the hips turn left and right over the feet, which remain where they are on the floor.

Let your attention move slowly up your body to your shoulders. As you turn to the left, the left shoulder moves backward and the right shoulder moves forward. Then, as you turn back to the right, the right shoulder moves backward and the left shoulder moves forward.

Bring your attention up to your head. Let your head turn to the left and right, along with the rest of the body; as you turn to the right, your chin should approach your right shoulder, and as you turn to the left, your chin should approach your left shoulder.

Continue to turn to the left and right like this, letting the whole body move in an easy, turning motion. Let the arms swing easily so that they make contact with the body in front and back as you come to the maximum turning angle on each side.

After a few minutes of turning in this manner, continue to turn, but reverse the motion of the head. (Photos 7-3, 7-4) As the hips and shoulders turn to the left, turn your head to the right so that the chin approaches the right shoulder. Then, as the hips and shoulders turn to the right, turn the head to the left so that the chin approaches the left shoulder. Make about 25 repetitions of this motion and again turn the head along with the body. Can you see that the turning angle of the body has increased?

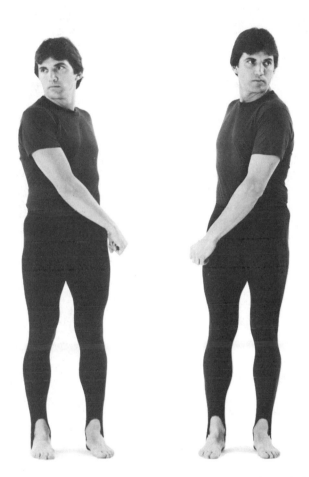

Photos 7-3, 7-4: *Now turn your whole body left and right while you turn your head in the opposite direction.*

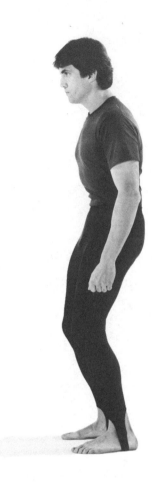

Photo 7-5: *Slowly bend your knees a little so that your head moves down a few inches.*

After you have spent a few minutes turning, stop and just stand still. Slowly bend your knees a little and then straighten them. (Photo 7-5) Bend your knees just enough so that your head moves about 5 or 6 inches down and then straighten them so that the head moves back up.

As you continue to do this, notice your ankle and hip joints. Both of these joints bend just enough so the feet remain flat on the floor and the torso remains vertical.

Now resume your turning motion, turning your body from left to right and back again. As you turn to the left, bend your knees a little, and as you turn back to the right, straighten them. (Photos 7-6, 7-7)

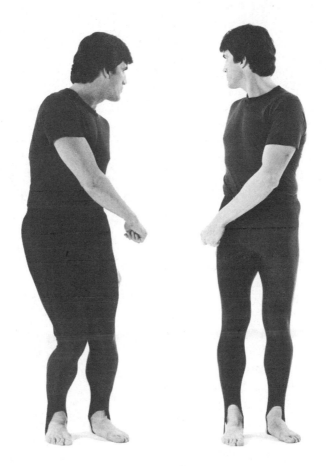

Photos 7-6, 7-7: *Turn your entire body—hips, shoulders, head, and eyes—to the left as you bend your knees a little. Then straighten your knees as you turn to the right.*

Continue to move in this way and scan your body from head to toe with your attention, as before. Notice every detail and compare the motion now with the initial turning motion, when you were not bending the knees. Does the bending of the knees interfere with the turning of the body at all? Can you still feel that your chin approaches first one shoulder and then the other as you turn left and right?

Spend a few minutes at this and then reverse the bending of the knees. As you turn to the right, bend your knees; as you turn to the left, straighten them. Again scan your body with your attention and make sure that the bending of the knees does not interfere with the turning motion of the body.

By moving with a simple, repetitive turning motion of the body like this and then bending and straightening the knees as we turn, we can discover if the motion of the knees affects the turning of the hips and shoulders. Many people stiffen their neck muscles and immobilize their heads or hold their breath when they begin to bend the knees; it usually requires several minutes of careful attention for them to become aware of this constriction of their motion. They probably do the same thing when running, but are unaware of it.

Rest for a minute and then resume the turning motion of the body. As you turn to each side, bend the knees, then straighten them when you are in the middle of the turn. As you rotate left and right, you will be bobbing up and down. When you face left or right, your knees will be bent and your head will be lower. When you face the middle, your knees will be straight and your head will be higher. Continue to move in this way and again scan your body, head to toe. Does this different motion of the knees interfere with the turning motion of the body?

As you continue to turn, straighten the knees as you turn to each side and bend them when you are in the middle. Spend a few minutes at this, then stop and rest. Walk around a little and swing your hips and shoulders. How does your walk feel?

When we walk or run, of course, we rotate our hips and shoulders in opposite directions, not in the same

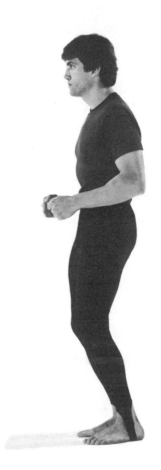

Photo 7-8: *Bend your knees slightly and also bend your elbows so that your fore-arms are almost horizontal.*

direction as we have been doing so far. So now let's begin to rotate the hips and shoulders in opposite directions.

Again stand with your feet about shoulder-width apart. Bend your knees very slightly and also bend your elbows so that your forearms are almost horizontal. (Photo 7-8) From this position, begin to rotate your hips and shoulders in opposite directions. (Photo 7-9) As the

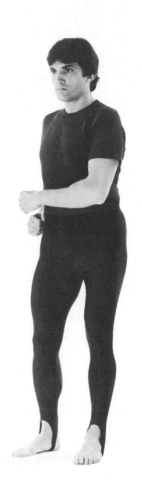

Photo 7-9: *With your knees still bent slightly, rotate your hips and shoulders in opposite directions.*

right hip moves back, the right shoulder moves forward, the left hip moves forward, and the left shoulder moves back.

Continue to move like this and scan your body as before. Notice your toes and the rest of your feet, and your legs, hips, torso, and shoulders. What are you doing with your head? Is it still or is it turning left and right? Notice your breathing. Do you hold your breath as you do the motion?

Pay careful attention to your hips and shoulders. Are they really moving in opposite directions? You'll probably find that the hips move quite a bit and that the shoulders

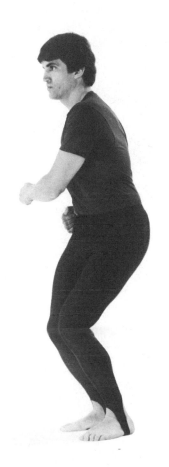

Photo 7-10: *With your knees bent, rotate your hips to the left and your shoulders to the right. Then straighten your knees and let your hips and shoulders return to center.*

move only a little, like the old dance called "the twist."

Spend a few minutes at this, getting a clear feeling for the motion of the hips and shoulders. Then add the bending and straightening of the knees to the motion.

Moving very slowly, so that you can pay attention to all details, rotate the hips to the left and the shoulders to the right, and at the same time bend the knees a little bit. (Photo 7-10) Then reverse the motion, straighten the knees, and let the hips and shoulders return to center. Repeat this motion many times and slowly scan your body as before. Do you find that the motion is easier when you think about one part of your body and not so easy when

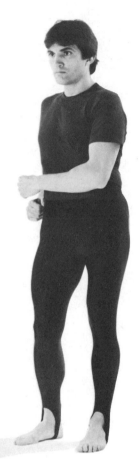 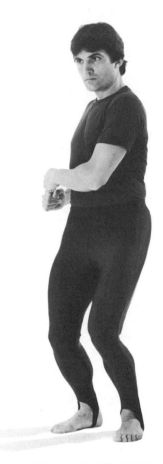

Photo 7-11: *Rotate your hips to the left and your shoulders to the right (Count 1).*

Photo 7-12: *With your hips still rotated left and your shoulders right, bend your knees (Count 2).*

you think about another? The parts where the motion is more difficult are the parts where your awareness is poor.

Now, instead of stopping and reversing the motion, let's continue it. When you first try this motion, think of it as four separate counts. First, rotate the hips left and the shoulders right. (Photo 7-11) Second, bend the knees. (Photo 7-12) Third, rotate the hips right and the shoulders

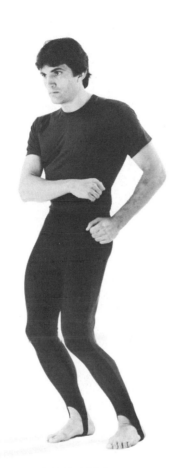 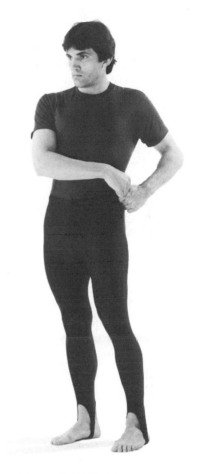

Photo 7-13: *With your knees still bent, rotate your hips right and your shoulders left (Count 3).*

Photo 7-14: *Now straighten your knees (Count 4). Repeat the entire sequence starting with Count 1.*

left. (Photo 7-13) Fourth, straighten the knees. (Photo 7-14) Then repeat the first move, rotating the hips left and the shoulders right, bend the knees again, and continue on.

As you move, make each motion clear and distinct. When you are moving the knees on counts two and four, do not move the hips and shoulders. Then, on counts one and three, when you are moving the hips and shoulders, do not change the angle of the knees.

Continue to move like this and slowly scan your body as before. When the move becomes clear, you can begin to speed it up just a little. Notice how, if you just let your body learn the move without hurrying, the movement gradually becomes easy to do; and at a certain point, you can "let go" of the motion, and the hips, shoulders, and knees will begin to move in a smooth, circular kind of movement that has a nice, coordinated feeling.

Spend a few minutes doing this and then reverse the direction and go the other way. Begin slowly, as before. First, rotate the hips right and the shoulders left. Second, bend the knees. Third, rotate the hips left and the shoulders right. Fourth, straighten the knees. Then repeat the first move, rotating the hips right and the shoulders left, and continue on. Try the move going in this direction for a few minutes and then go back and try the initial direction again.

If you have difficulty with this motion, do not try to force yourself to do it right away. Instead, spend 10 or 15 minutes at it, forget about it for a few days, then try it again. You'll be surprised at how much easier it is after a little time has passed. What kind of learning process is going on inside you to make the move easier without any effort on your part?

When you can do this move easily, demonstrate it for a friend and ask him to copy the move. He will almost certainly be unable to do it without going through the process you just went through in order to learn it. What does this tell you about the value of just trying to copy the motions of someone else—like an expert runner—when you're trying to learn something?

When you have finished with this lesson, walk around a little and notice the smooth, coordinated feeling in the hips and shoulders. You may even feel a bounce in your walk that wasn't there before. All of this comes from your increased awareness of the motions of the hips and shoulders, and how those motions interact with the bending of the knees.

Learning to move the hips, shoulders, and legs like this can improve your running dramatically. This pattern of movement activates combinations of motion in these three parts of the body that many people never use. The resulting freedom of movement will affect your running in a very positive way.

Marta: One-Step Learning

When Marta came to talk to me about my running class, she had a very strange request. "I want to take your class—or at least I think I do—but I don't want to run."

I stared at Marta for about 10 seconds trying to think of something to say. Finally, I managed to get out a "Huh?"

She repeated her question and watched me patiently for another 10 seconds while I stared at her some more. Finally I managed to think of a more elaborate reply. "But running is what the class is all about!"

"I have been talking to a couple of friends of mine," Marta continued, unfazed. "They told me that most of the class is about walking, and that's what I want to do."

"Well, yes, we do a lot of walking in the class, but as I recall, you walked in here without much trouble. What's wrong with your walking?" I asked.

"Well, I don't have any trouble just walking around, but I like to take long walks—or at least I used to. A few months ago my right knee started to hurt a lot whenever I went more than a mile or two, and now I can't go nearly as far as I like. Do you think your class could help?"

"Well, it probably could," I told her. "But tell me a little more. Have you ever injured your knee?"

Marta and I had a long talk about walking and running. She was slim, attractive, and turned out to be quite a bit older than the 40 years that I had guessed her age to be. Marta became very enthusiastic about the class as we talked. It was pretty obvious that she missed her long walks a lot.

On the first day of class, Marta paid very careful attention as I directed everyone to feel how their hips and shoulders moved as they advanced first one foot and then the other. Marta seemed to have a little more trouble getting into the motions than the others in the class, but in the end she was able to exaggerate the hip and shoulder motion or to lock the hips and shoulders together without much effort. Marta concentrated intently on the motions and asked more questions than the rest of the class put together. I could see that she was determined to succeed and I really wanted to help her. At the conclusion of the first session, Marta seemed really pleased and thanked me profusely.

I was kind of surprised, then, when Marta didn't show up for the next session, or the next; the *only* class she attended, in fact, was the first. I ran into some mutual friends and asked if she was ill. They told me that she was working, and as far as they knew, she was fine.

I couldn't understand it. Marta had seemed so pleased after the first session, and then she had just dropped out. I thought about her off and on for months. It really bothered me that she had started the class with such enthusiasm and then just stopped attending without explanation. I wondered what had happened. And then one day I ran into her while shopping.

"Hi," I said, "remember me?"

"Well, of course I remember you," she replied. "You know, I can't thank you enough for that running class. It was just marvelous."

"Well . . . if you liked it so much, why didn't you come back after the first time?"

"I told you that I didn't want to run."

"I guess I still don't understand. We don't start running until the very end, and you stopped coming after the first class."

"But all I wanted was to be able to go back to my long walks without my knee hurting."

Finally it hit me. "You mean you got it after that one class?" I asked. "Your knee stopped hurting after just one class?"

"That's right," Marta said. "I went out the very next day, and walked about 5 miles. I just kept swinging my hips and shoulders like you said, and my knee never bothered me at all."

"Actually, there's a lot more to it than that," I started, but she was looking at her watch. "I have to be going now," she said, "so goodbye, and thank you again."

After she walked away, I thought about her and her pain, and about how easy it had been to help her by giving her just a simple understanding of the principles of human learning and movement.

Then I thought back to some of the other people I had helped. Some, like Naomi, had just taken a few minutes, and I thought about the precision and power of a method that can produce such results in such a short time.

Then I thought back even further, many years back, and I remembered a teenager with a painful right knee. I remembered that one fine spring Saturday that he had played football from about noon until early evening, when his knee had become so painful and swollen that his mother had had to cut his pants off with a pair of scissors.

A few days later the swelling was gone and the usual specialists had been consulted. A careful examination revealed no cause for the boy's pain, and so a high-quality, well-fitting shoe had been prescribed for everyday wear. This should eliminate problems with the knee, he had been told, as long as he stayed away from football and too much running.

As I thought of that boy, I wished that I could go back and tell him what I know now, explain to him that he didn't really have a weak body or a defective knee. I wished I could tell him that it was just a matter of changing the way he moved a little, and then he could have run and jumped just as much as anyone else.

But then, I thought, he would never have written this book.

8

Shoulders, Spine, and Hips

For your hips and shoulders to move in a smooth, coordinated way when you are running, your spine must be able to move easily. The hips, of course, are strongly connected to the spine. For one hip to rise up toward the head, the spine must be able to curve to the side. And for the hip to move forward, the spine must be able to rotate.

When running, the hip over the advancing foot moves forward and up; as it does, the spine must bend and rotate in a very complex motion if the hip is to move easily. If some parts of your spine are stiff, they will restrict the motion of your hips and throw off your running.

Although the connection between the spine and the hips—through the bones of the sacrum—is very direct, the connections between the shoulders and the spine are more indirect. The only bony connections between the shoulders and the spine are through the collarbone to the sternum, then through the ribs, and finally to the spine. Because of this, the shoulders have a much wider range of motion than the hips and they can move relatively

independently of the spine. Nevertheless, the mobility of
the spine also strongly affects the mobility and ease of
movement of the shoulders.

In this chapter we're going to explore some of these
connections between the spine, hips, and shoulders. As
you begin to feel how the spine works in conjunction with
the hips and shoulders to allow them to move easily, you
will find that the movements of your hips and shoulders
improve in such a way that your running becomes much
easier and freer.

Sit down and lean back on your hands, elbows
straight. Put the soles of your feet together and draw
them in close to your body, with your knees opened out.
Slide your feet out a little bit away from you and then back
in closer a few times, until you find a place for the feet that
feels comfortable. (Photo 8-1)

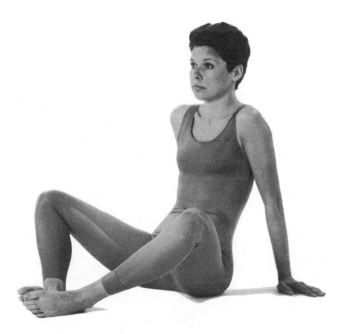

Photo 8-1: *Sit down and lean back on your hands, elbows
straight. Put the soles of your feet together and draw them in
comfortably close to your body.*

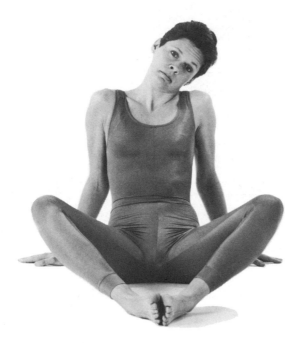

Photo 8-2: *Tilt your head to the left so that your left ear approaches your left shoulder.*

Slowly move your left ear toward your left shoulder. Tilt your head as far as is easy to the left and then come back to center. (Photo 8-2) Repeat this motion 25 times and notice if you feel anything in your spine and hips as you move. After 25 repetitions, stop, lie on your back, and rest. Notice how your upper body touches the floor. Can you feel any difference between the left and right sides?

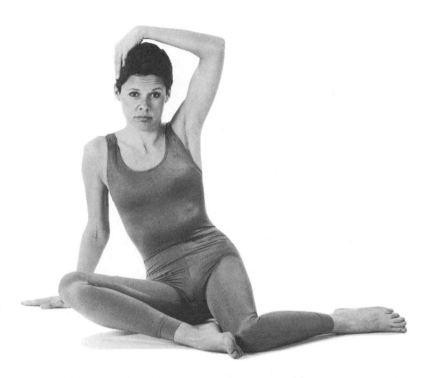

Photo 8-3: *Change your position so that your left knee is near your right foot, and put your left hand on top of your head, fingertips touching your right ear.*

Roll to one side and sit up, lean back on your hands, and draw in your feet so that the soles touch. Pick up your left leg and turn it over on the floor so that the left knee is close to the right foot and the left foot is near the left buttock. Put the palm of your left hand on top of your head with the left elbow pointing out to the side. (Photo 8-3)

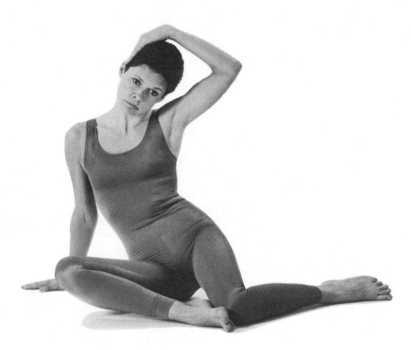

Photo 8-4: *Let your head and left arm drop to the left side together and then bring them back up.*

From this position, let the head and left arm drop to the side together and then raise them back up. (Photo 8-4) Repeat this motion 25 times, noticing how the spine curves to the side as the head drops to the left.

Stop moving, replace the left hand on the floor behind you, and turn the left leg over on the floor so that the soles of the feet are touching again. Drop the head to the left a few times, letting the left ear approach the left shoulder as you did earlier. Notice how the head moves farther and more easily now. Stop moving, lie on your back, and rest.

Once again, roll to one side and sit up. Place the soles of your feet together with your knees opened out and lean back on your hands. From this position, drop the right knee down toward the floor and then let it come back to its starting position. (Photo 8-5) Continue this motion and

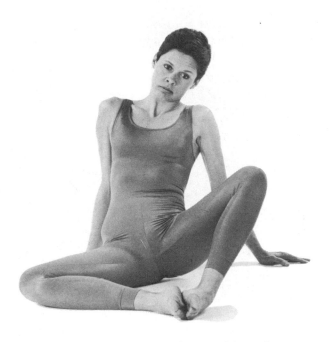

Photo 8-5: *Return to your starting position; then move your right knee down toward the floor.*

notice what you do with the rest of your body to let the right knee drop. Can you feel the weight shift onto your right buttock as you do this? Pay attention to your hands on the floor. Can you feel that one hand presses into the floor more than the other as the knee drops? Can you feel that your spine moves in some way as the knee goes down? Make about 25 repetitions of the motion and then stop.

Once again, move your left ear toward your left shoulder as you did just a minute ago. Does the head move a little more easily to the side now? Lie on your back and rest.

Roll to one side and sit up, soles of the feet touching, knees out, and lean back on your hands. Notice the distance between your left ribs and your left elbow. Move the ribs on your left side to the right so that they move away from the left elbow a little bit, and then let them

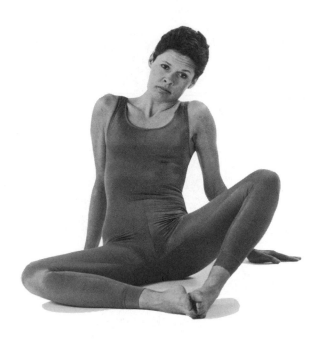

Photo 8-6: *Move the ribs on your left side to the right so that they move away from your left elbow a little bit.*

come back to the resting position. (Photo 8-6) Repeat this motion and notice how the spine must move in back to allow the ribs to move away from the elbow. As you move, let your attention go up and down your spine. Does the whole spine curve gently to the side to allow the ribs to move, or are there stiff areas, or places that your awareness does not reach?

Continue to move and notice how the pressure of your buttocks on the floor moves over to the right side, and how the right knee drops down toward the floor, as the ribs move away from the elbow on the left side. Let your left ear approach your left shoulder as the ribs move away and the right knee drops down.

As you move like this, imagine that the spine curves to the right like a "")'' when seen from behind, to make the ribs on the left side move away from the elbow. As the spine curves, the head tilts to the left so that the left ear approaches the left shoulder and the pelvis tilts so that the right knee drops down closer to the floor.

Pay attention to one aspect of the motion, such as the knee or the head, and then think of another aspect, and another, until you get the feeling that all of the individual moves—the head, the knee, the ribs, the hand pushing on the floor, the pelvis tilting—are actually all parts of one big move, which is the spine curving to the side. The spine is the conductor of the orchestra of the head, ribs, pelvis, knees, and hands. If the spine does its job correctly, all these parts will move in a coordinated, harmonious way. If the spine is not well organized, the parts move in a jerky, uncoordinated fashion.

After at least 25 repetitions of the movement, stop, lie on your back, and rest. Compare the feeling in the left and right sides of the body and notice how the shoulders, back, and hips touch the floor on the left and right side.

Roll to one side and sit up, soles of the feet touching, and lean back on your hands. Begin to move your right ear toward your right shoulder. Let the ear drop as close to the shoulder as is easy and then bring the head back to center. Repeat this motion 25 times and notice what happens in the rest of your spine as you tilt your head to the right. Stop, lie down, and rest.

Roll over and sit up with the soles of your feet touching, knees opened, and lean back on your hands behind you. Pick up your right leg and turn it over on the floor so that the right knee is close to the left foot and the right foot is close to the right buttock. Place the palm of your right hand on top of your head so that the right elbow is facing to the right.

From this position, tilt the head and right arm to the right so that the right elbow drops down toward the floor; then return the head and arm to the center. Repeat this move slowly about 25 times and notice just where the spine curves in back to allow the head and arm to drop down.

Now replace the right hand on the floor behind you and turn the right leg over on the floor so that the soles of the feet are touching. Once again, tilt the head to the right so that the right ear approaches the right shoulder, then bring the head back to center. Repeat this motion a few times and notice how the head moves farther and more easily. Lie on your back and rest.

Again sit up with the soles of your feet touching and lean back on your hands behind you. Move your left knee down toward the floor as far as is easy and then let it come back to its resting position. Continue to move the left knee down and up and notice how your weight shifts over to your left buttock and how the right hand pushes into the floor. Pay attention to the distance between the ribs on the right side and the right elbow. Do the ribs move away from the elbow as the knee drops down? Make 25 repetitions of this motion and then lie down and rest on your back for a minute.

Roll over and sit up as before. Move the right ribs away from the right elbow. Move the ribs to the left a little and then let them come back to their initial position. Continue to move the ribs and notice how the whole spine must curve to the left to allow the ribs to move. As the spine curves to the left, of course, the two ends of the spine—the head and the hips—must move. Notice how the head tilts to the right so that the right ear approaches the right shoulder, how the pelvis tilts on the floor so that the pressure moves over to the left buttock, and how the left knee drops toward the floor. Make 25 or more repetitions of the motion, until all parts of the movement are clear, and then lie down and rest.

Again sit up with the soles of the feet touching and lean back on your hands. Tilt your head to the left so that the left ear approaches the left shoulder, and then tilt the head to the right so that the right ear approaches the right shoulder. Continue to tilt the head left and right like this, letting the rest of the body follow the move so that first one hand and then the other pushes on the floor. The weight should shift from the left to the right buttock and back, and the knees should rise and fall toward the floor.

Pay particular attention to how the spine curves in back and how first one side of the body and then the other becomes shorter as the spine curves. As the right ear approaches the right shoulder, the ribs on the right side are compressed and the right knee rises as if to meet the right ear. Then, as the head tilts to the left, the left side gets compressed and the right side elongates. Make 25 repetitions of this motion and then lie down and rest. Notice how your body makes contact with the floor. Pay particular attention to your spine. Can you feel exactly where the whole spine is located?

Sit up again, soles of the feet touching, and lean back on your hands. Let your head drop forward so that your chin is close to your chest. (Photo 8-7) From this position, push your stomach out so that it gets round in front. (Photo 8-8) Then let it drop back to its resting position. Continue to do this and notice how the pelvis rolls forward so that the pressure shifts toward the front of the pelvis on the floor, and how the curve in the small of the back increases as the stomach protrudes. Also notice how the ribs move away from the elbows and how the chin rises up

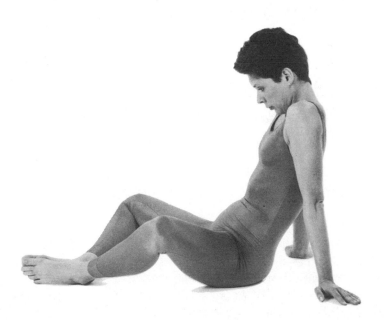

Photo 8-7: *Drop your head forward so that your chin approaches your chest.*

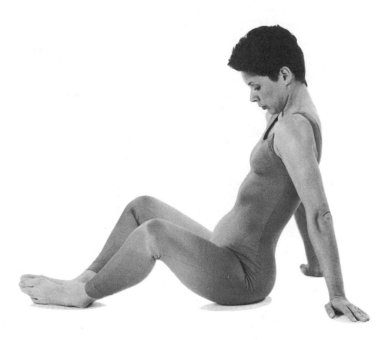

Photo 8-8: *Letting the head hang down, push your stomach out so that your pelvis rolls forward on the floor.*

off the chest a little—in short, how the whole spine moves as the stomach is pushed out and the pelvis rolls forward on the floor.

Make 25 repetitions of this motion and let your attention move up your spine from your pelvis through the small of the back, on up between the shoulder blades, and through the neck to the head. If you make small, slow, easy motions and don't try to push yourself to the limit of your ability, you'll be able to feel which parts of the spine move and which do not.

Sit straight up, take the weight off your hands for a minute, and rest. Then lean back on your hands again and let your head drop backward so that the chin is far away from the chest. (Photo 8-9) From this position, again push the stomach out and let the pelvis roll forward, then let the stomach come back to its resting position. (Photo 8-10) Continue to move and notice how the motion of the

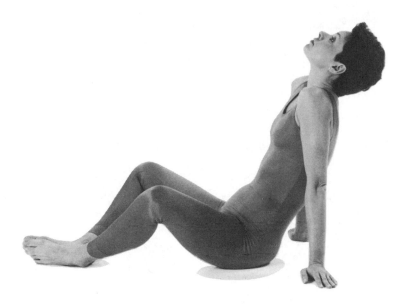

Photo 8-9: *Now drop your head back so that your chin moves up and away from your chest.*

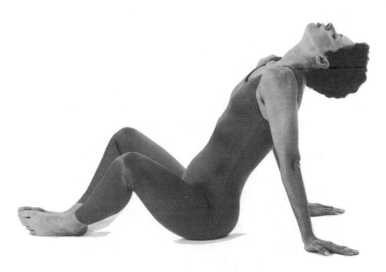

Photo 8-10: *With your head hanging back, push your stomach out so that your pelvis rolls forward on the floor.*

spine is transmitted up through the neck to the head so that the head drops back even farther as the stomach is pushed out. Make another 25 repetitions, then bring your head up to its usual position, so that you are looking straight ahead, and continue to move. Can you still feel that the motion of the spine goes all the way up to the head, so that the head nods up and down a little as the stomach is pushed out and back? Lie on your back and rest.

Roll over and sit up, soles of the feet touching, and lean back on your hands. Push your stomach out and let your pelvis roll forward. Then pull your stomach in, rounding your back and letting your pelvis roll on the floor so that your weight shifts back toward your tailbone. Continue to move in this way and scan your body with your attention, carefully noting all the details of the motion. Notice how your hands push on the floor to help the pelvis roll forward and how the ribs move away from the elbows.

Think of the whole spine curving in back, becoming concave as you push your stomach out and then convex as the stomach is pulled in. (Photos 8-11, 8-12) As the ribs move away from the elbows, the head tilts back so that you look up; then, as the ribs come closer to the elbows, the head tilts forward so that you look down. Check your breathing. Is it slow and even? Make 25 or more repetitions of this motion, until all the details are clear, and then lie down and rest.

Once more sit up with the soles of your feet touching and lean back on your hands. Bend your spine left and right as you did earlier, letting the pelvis and head tilt to the sides. Notice the point of contact between the pelvis and the floor. As the pelvis tilts left and right, the point of maximum pressure shifts in a line from the left to the right side of the pelvis, drawing a straight line on the floor. Stop moving your spine from side to side and bend it forward and back, so that the pelvis rolls forward and back on the floor and the head nods up and down. Again, notice the point of contact of the pelvis and the floor. This time the point of contact draws a straight line at right angles to the

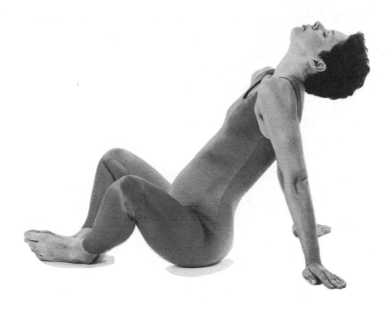

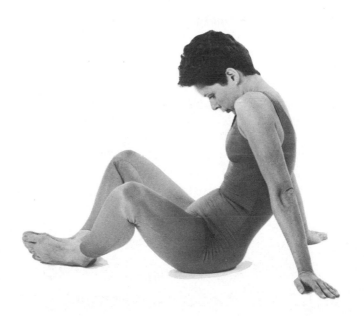

Photos 8-11, 8-12: *Push your stomach out, rotating your pelvis forward on the floor, then pull your stomach in, so that the pelvis rolls back on the floor.*

first line, moving from the front to the back of the pelvis.

Move your pelvis forward and back and left and right a number of times, until you have a clear picture of the two lines and how they form a cross, with the center of the cross in the middle of the pelvis as it rests on the floor. When you are clear about the two lines, begin to draw a circle on the floor around the center of the cross by moving the pelvis. Move slowly so that you can allow the rest of the body to follow along.

As you draw the circle, let your attention move through your body. Notice how your spine and ribs move, and how first one hand presses into the floor and then the other. Pay attention to the motion of the knees and notice how the head moves in a combination of the side-to-side and front-to-back tilting motions it was making earlier. Make 25 repetitions of the circles in one direction, making sure that you breathe easily, and then reverse the direction and make another 25 circles the other way. When you're finished, lie down and rest.

As you lie there, check the contact of your back with the floor. Pay particular attention to your pelvis, spine, and head. Can you feel exactly where each of these parts is located with respect to the others and in relation to the floor?

Roll over to one side and stand up. How does it feel to stand? Walk around a little and swing your hips and shoulders as you walk. Think of your spine as you move. Can you feel your spine moving as you swing your hips and shoulders? Notice how much easier and more coordinated the motion of the hips and shoulders feels now that the spine is involved in the motion.

Mike: Does Running Have to Be Difficult?

Sometimes after my running classes there is a little extra time, and I invite questions. Usually the questions are pretty straightforward and I don't have much trouble answering them. Every once in a while, though, someone asks a question that I've never thought about, and the answer turns out to be pretty interesting.

This happened once toward the end of a class. Everyone was sitting in a circle, just talking about running. I could see Mike, a quiet man in his late 20s, working up the nerve to say something; Mike had gone through the whole class without speaking once. Now he shifted his position, cleared his throat nervously, looked around, and finally said, "Can I ask a question?"

"Sure," I said, "fire away."

"Well," Mike began hesitantly, "I'm not sure that I know just how to say this. Anyway, it will probably sound kind of strange.

"I've been running a little between the classes and working on the things that we've learned, and it's really made a big difference in my running. It's faster and smoother, and my breathing is better, but . . . well, it's just too *easy* to run now. It doesn't feel *right*," he blurted out. The whole class laughed, and Mike's face turned red.

"But that's what we've been working toward all along," I said.

"I know that, and it sounds like just what I need, but it doesn't feel anything like I thought it would feel," he said. "It's kind of a letdown. I expected it to be a lot harder."

"Does anybody else feel that way?" I asked.

A few other people raised their hands, and someone said, "Yeah, sort of."

I asked the class to give me a minute to think about the question before I answered. At first I thought that Mike's question was kind of dumb. He was complaining about the very thing he had come to the class for, the very thing that I had said I was going to teach in the class.

But all of a sudden I remembered a few years back, when I had taught myself downhill skiing. After years of struggling to learn to ski, I had finally figured out how to do it and I had had an incredible breakthrough in my skiing. I remembered distinctly thinking at the time that skiing had suddenly become too easy. It wasn't a challenge anymore. My skis had suddenly learned to turn by themselves, or so it seemed. At that point I decided that maybe Mike's question wasn't so dumb after all, and I thought long and hard before answering it.

"In our society, we teach ourselves to expect learning to be difficult," I began. "It's always 'Work *hard* and you'll succeed,' or 'Try *harder* and you'll get it.' So after a few years of that we begin to get the feeling that if we don't have to kill ourselves to do something, it's not really worthwhile. We become so used to struggling to accomplish our goals that we learn to equate the feeling of more effort with better performance—when it should be just the opposite.

"That idea of 'more effort equals better performance' gets right down into our bones and muscles, too. We have all walked and run for years and we each have certain sensations in the muscles of the legs and body that tell us if we are moving correctly—or what we think of as correctly. When that sensation starts to change, it feels very peculiar, almost as if we have lost a part of ourselves.

"As a result, when we finally begin to do something with a little skill, it usually doesn't feel right at first."

"So what can we do about that?" Mike asked.

"I don't have a quick-fix for that problem," I told Mike. "It's just something that you have to experiment with and think about and find out for yourself. But you must have the basic idea already, or you wouldn't have asked the question that you did."

The class had been following our discussion carefully, and now everyone suddenly started talking at once. Half of them seemed to agree with me and the other half disagreed. One man said that he had several friends who just about killed themselves running and yet they managed to win some races. Furthermore, he said, they enjoyed putting out the effort, or at least they claimed they did. An older man chimed in that he also had known people like that 15 years ago—and now they all had knee problems.

Finally the question came back to me again. I felt as if I hadn't made my point.

"Let me put it this way," I said. "My idea is that you

can learn to run with the same kind of quality that some people have when they play a musical instrument. You can't use force to play well because you'll only get more volume, not better music. So you have to experiment with timing, and learn just how to place your fingers on the keys, or strings, or whatever, and if you persist, you can learn to play. What I'm trying to do here is to teach you to learn to move with that kind of quality. To 'play your body,' if you want to call it that. Does that answer your question?"

Mike thought about what I had said. "I guess so," he said. "It really does feel good to run this new way, and what you said makes a lot of sense. I suppose anything new and different just takes some time to get used to."

9

The
Motion
of the Feet

When we run, each foot comes down onto the ground and takes our entire weight with every step. The foot is able to survive this kind of punishment because it is a true marvel of biological engineering. The foot doesn't do its job alone, however. For the foot to work properly, the ankle joint, the bones of the lower leg, and the knee and hip joints all have to work in concert with the foot.

For many people, the foot doesn't work as well as it should. A few miles of running or just an unusual amount of time spent walking around, as on a day of sightseeing, produces pain in the feet. Usually it's not just the foot itself that is at fault in these cases, but rather the way that the foot works—or doesn't work—with the ankle, knee, and hip joints.

As the foot comes down onto the ground to take a step, it moves and flattens out so that the force is equally distributed throughout the foot and no one part is subjected to a disproportionate amount of force. For this to happen, the ankle and hip joints must work together in a particular way. It is this connection between the foot and the hip that we're going to explore and improve in this chapter.

120

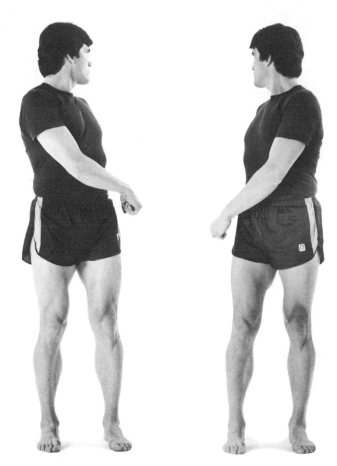

Photos 9-1, 9-2: *Stand in your normal standing posture and turn your whole body left and right; make sure your head turns left and right over your shoulders.*

Take off your shoes and socks and put on a pair of shorts so that you can clearly see your feet, ankles, and legs. Stand in your normal standing posture and turn your whole body left and right in an easy, twisting motion. (Photos 9-1, 9-2) Make sure the head turns left and right over the shoulders so that the chin approaches the left shoulder as you turn left and the right shoulder as you turn right.

As you turn, direct your attention to the bottoms of your feet. Begin with the right foot. Notice how it tilts on the floor as the body turns. When you turn to the right, the right foot tilts so that its outside edge presses into the floor, and when you turn to the left, it tilts in the opposite direction so that the inside edge presses into the floor.

Continue to turn left and right like this, paying careful attention to the right foot. Notice that as you turn to the right and the weight shifts to the outside edge, the foot moves so that the arch increases and the toes come a little closer to the heel. Then, as you turn to the left and the pressure shifts to the inside edge, the arch decreases and the toes move away from the heel.

As you turn left and right like this, exaggerate the motion of the right foot so that as you turn to the left, the foot tilts far to the left and the arch completely flattens out on the floor, and as you turn to the right, the foot tilts to the right and the arch rises up high. (Photos 9-3, 9-4)

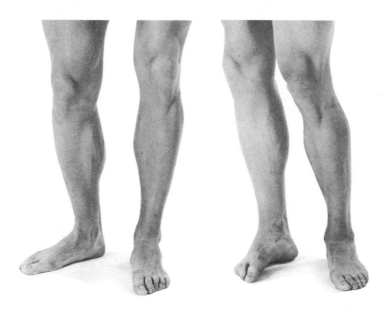

Photos 9-3, 9-4: *Exaggerate the motion of your right foot so that as you turn to the left, the arch flattens out on the floor, and as you turn to the right, the arch rises up high.*

Make 25 or more moves like this, then stop and rest for a minute.

Standing as before, turn your whole body left and right. As you turn, compare the feeling in your left and right feet. Do the two feet feel as if they are moving differently? Now turn to the right and stop with your whole body facing right. (Photo 9-5) From this position,

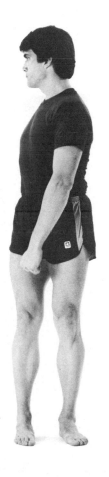

Photo 9-5: *Now turn to the right and stop, with your whole body facing to the right.*

tilt the right foot right and left on the floor. (Photos 9-6, 9-7) Look down at the foot so that you can see how it's moving. Make sure that as the outside edge of the right foot presses into the floor, the arch rises up. As the right foot tilts left and the inside edge presses down, the arch should flatten out on the floor.

Continue to tilt the foot left and right like this and observe your right leg. Notice how the leg rotates as the foot tilts. Follow this rotation up your leg to your knee, which should be straight, and then to your hip joint. Can you feel the hip joint moving? The muscles that tilt the foot left and right are actually the muscles around the hip joint. If the muscles here are tight, the foot may not be able to flatten out on the ground easily when you take a step, and you could develop pains or injuries in the foot. Make at least 25 tilting motions of the right foot and then swing

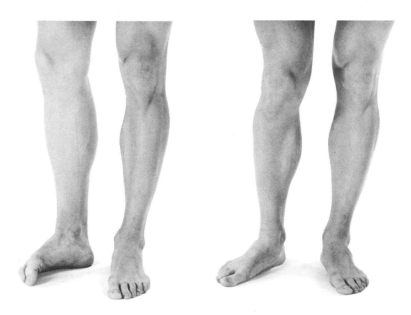

Photos 9-6, 9-7: *With your body facing right, tilt your right foot right and left on the floor. Look down at your foot so that you can see how it is moving.*

your body left and right as before. After a few turns, turn all the way to the left and stop. Once again, tilt the right foot left and right on the floor as you just did. Again notice how the right leg rotates left and right to tilt the foot. After about 25 movements of the foot, go back to turning the whole body and compare the feeling in the two feet. Which foot feels as though it's moving better on the floor? Stop turning and rest for a minute.

Again turn your body left and right, as you have been doing. Turn to the left, letting the right foot tilt so that its inside edge presses into the floor and the arch flattens out, and stop. (Photo 9-8) Hold the right foot in this

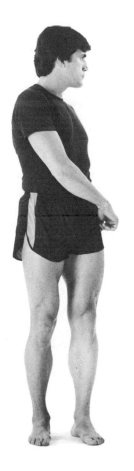

Photo 9-8: *Turn to the left, letting your right foot tilt so that the arch flattens out, and stop.*

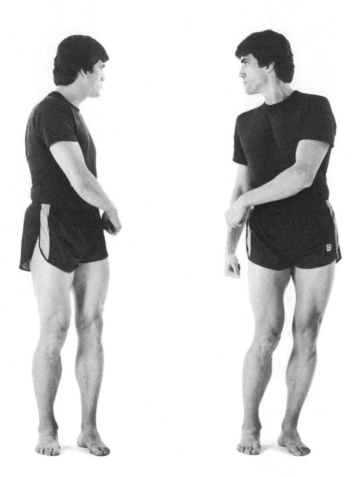

Photos 9-9, 9-10: *Holding your right foot immobile, turn your body left and right. Notice how holding your foot still will restrict the turning angle to the right.*

position and turn your body left and right. (Photos 9-9, 9-10) Holding the foot still like this will restrict the turning angle to the right. Turn your body only as far as is easy to each side and then come back. Make 25 turns, release the right foot, and continue to turn your body left and right. Notice how the two feet move on the floor. Which moves more easily? Stop turning and walk around a little. Pay careful attention to each foot as it contacts the floor. Can you identify the difference between the two feet? Stop and rest for a minute.

Once again, turn your body left and right. This time, focus your attention on your left foot. Notice how the left foot tilts left and right on the floor as the body turns. As you turn to the left, the weight shifts to the outside edge of the foot and the arch of the foot rises up. As you turn to the right, the weight shifts to the inside edge of the foot and the arch flattens out.

Continue turning left and right and exaggerate the motions of the left foot as you did earlier with the right foot. As you do this, look down at your foot so that you can see and feel how the foot and ankle move.

After 25 or more repetitions, turn to the left and stop, with the weight shifted to the outside of the left foot and the arch of the left foot up. Holding the body turned to the left, tilt the left foot left and right on the floor by rotating the left leg left and right, as you did before with the right leg. Notice how the foot tilts on the floor and how the arch moves up and down. Make 25 repetitions while facing left and then turn to the right and make another 25 tilting movements of the left foot. Stop and rest for a minute.

Now turn left and right again. Make a few turns and then stop, with the body turned to the right and the left foot tilted to the right, so that all the pressure is on the inside of the foot and the arch is flat against the floor. Hold the foot in this position and turn the body left and right. Keeping the foot still like this will restrict the turning angle of the body. With this in mind, turn the body only so far as is easy. Make 25 turns and then stop. Release the foot and turn the whole body left and right. Direct your attention to the feet and compare the feeling of the feet moving against the floor with the way they felt at the beginning of this exercise.

Stop turning and face straight forward. (Photo 9-11) Keeping your body still, rotate both legs inward together so that both arches flatten out and the pressure shifts to the inside of the feet. Then rotate the legs outward so that

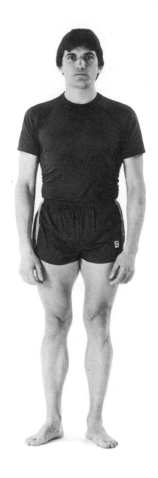

Photo 9-11: *Stop turning and face straight forward.*

both arches rise up and the pressure shifts to the outside of the feet. (Photos 9-12, 9-13) Continue to do this and look down at your feet so that you can see how they move. Notice that by rotating your hip joints you can give yourself flat feet or unusually high arches, as you wish.

Stop after about 25 repetitions, with your weight shifted to the outside edges of your feet and your arches high. Holding this position, flex and extend your toes. (Photos 9-14, 9-15) Push your toes down into the floor about 15 times and then raise them up off the floor; make sure that you do not hold your breath as you do this.

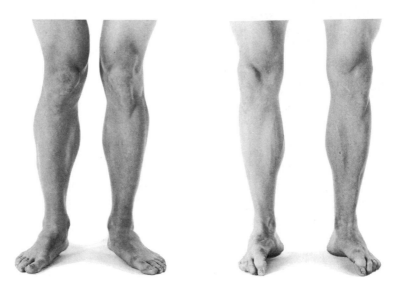

Photos 9-12, 9-13: *Rotate both legs inward together so that both arches flatten out; then rotate them outward so that both arches rise up.*

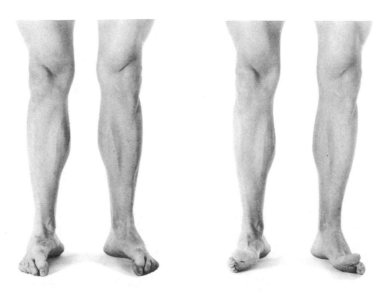

Photos 9-14, 9-15: *With your weight shifted to the outside edges of your feet and your arches high, push your toes into the floor and then raise them up off the floor.*

When you are finished, walk around a little. Notice how clear the sensation of the feet contacting the floor is and how softly and easily the feet come down onto the floor. Can you feel a sensation of fluidity and ease of motion in the hip joints also?

The next time you run, start off slowly and feel your feet coming down onto the ground. Gradually increase your speed and notice how your running is smoother, quicker, and more fluid than you have ever felt it.

Bif: Is the Problem Where the Pain Is?

After Bif completed my running class—and made his peace with his dog, Nicky—he really began to push his running. From 50 miles a week, he pushed up to about 80. Then, one day, I got a phone call.

"My left knee is killing me," he whimpered.

"Did you injure it?" I asked him.

"No," he said, "but the other day I ran 20 miles, and at the end of the run it hurt pretty badly. Now when I get up to 2 or 3 miles, it really hurts. It hurts so much I have to stop." It was a slow Saturday afternoon, so I asked Bif to come over to my house.

He brought a copy of Jim Fixx's running book with him. He showed me the section on runner's knee and asked me if I thought that was his problem. From the description in the book, it sounded as if that were it. What seemed strange to me, though, was why there was pain in only one knee. There had to be some difference between the left and right sides to cause pain in one knee and not the other. Bif agreed that my theory made sense, but he couldn't really feel a difference between the two sides.

After some more discussion, Bif asked if I thought his shoes could be causing the problem. He was wearing a good brand of shoes, but they were pretty worn.

"Let me see the bottoms of the shoes," I said.

Bif removed his shoes and gave them to me. I looked

at the wear pattern on the bottoms of Bif's shoes. On the right shoe, the heel area was well worn toward the outside and then the worn area continued up to the toes along the outside of the shoe. On the left shoe, however, the heel was worn down almost in the center and the wear pattern went straight up the middle of the shoe to the toes. I showed the two different wear patterns to Bif.

"You must be doing something very different with your left and right legs to produce such different wear patterns," I said. "Do you know what it is?"

Bif had no idea.

I asked him to walk back and forth across the floor without his shoes and to feel how the pressure moved along the bottom of each foot as he walked. Bif began to walk, concentrating on the sensations from his feet.

Suddenly he stopped walking. "Hey," he said, "I can feel it! On my right foot the pressure moves from the heel to the toes along the outside of the foot, but on the left foot it moves straight up the middle. I wonder why I never felt that before!"

I explained to Bif that when a foot is doing its job correctly, the heel strikes the ground first and then the pressure rolls around the outside of the foot and on up toward the toes, until the foot lifts up off the ground to take another step. His right foot was doing that, as proven by the wear pattern on the right shoe, but his left foot was not, and that showed just as clearly on the left shoe.

"Well, what are we going to do about it?" Bif asked.

"Stand here in front of me," I said, "with your feet about shoulder-width apart and turn your whole body left and right, but leave your feet where they are on the floor."

Bif began to swing his whole body left and right, and I sat down on the floor and watched his feet. As he turned to the right, his right foot tilted on the floor in such a way that the pressure shifted to the outside edge of the foot and the arch of the foot increased. As he turned to the left, the right foot tilted in the opposite direction so that the pressure moved to the inside edge of the foot, flattening the arch. The left foot, however, was almost immobile on the floor. It hardly moved at all as Bif turned left and right.

"Keep turning like you are," I said, "and look down at your feet and ankles. Look at the difference between the left and right sides."

"The right one's moving and the left one isn't," he said.

"That's right," I agreed, "and there's your problem, right there in that left ankle."

"Wait a second," said Bif. "The problem is in my left knee, not my left ankle."

"No, the *pain* is in your left knee, but the *problem* is in your left ankle."

Bif stopped turning and looked down at me. "I don't follow that at all," he said.

"Look," I said, "when you run, every time you take a step, about three times your whole weight comes down on each leg. Now, if all the joints are working properly, the force of the body coming down on the leg is distributed equally throughout the whole leg. But if one of the joints—like the ankle—isn't moving properly, some other joint—like the knee—has to take more force than it is designed to handle. And after a while it starts to hurt."

"I never thought of it that way," Bif admitted, "but it makes sense."

"Go back to that turning motion you were just doing," I said, "and let's get that left ankle going."

Bif began to turn left and right. "As you turn to the right," I said, "tilt your right foot on the floor so that the weight goes even more to the outside of the foot and increases the height of the arch, and when you turn to the left, tilt the foot so that the weight goes over to the inside of the foot and flattens the arch. In other words, just exaggerate the motion of the right foot."

"But I thought that we were going to work on the left ankle," Bif complained.

"We'll get there," I said. "Trust me."

Bif continued to turn left and right, exaggerating the motion of the right foot on the floor. I had him do a number of different moves with the right foot, such as turning his body left and right with the ankle and foot held still, and then tilting his foot left and right with his body held still. After about 30 minutes of this I asked Bif just to turn left and right without doing anything special with his feet. I could see that the right ankle and foot were turning along with the body even more than before and that the left ankle had started to move a little also. I pointed all this out to Bif.

"How come the left ankle changed when all the work that we did was with the right?" he asked.

"I guess the left ankle was listening while I was talking to the right one," I answered. "Now go back to that turning motion and let's do the whole thing over again with the left ankle."

After having had the experience of making all those strange moves with his right ankle, which was moving fairly well to begin with, it was simple for him to do it all over again on the left side.

As we were working with the motion of the left ankle and leg, Bif suddenly stopped turning and winced.

"What happened?" I asked.

"It feels like something moved about halfway up my spine over here on the left side," Bif answered. "It didn't really hurt that much, but it kind of caught me by surprise."

"Go back to that turning motion," I said, "I want to see something."

Bif began turning left and right again. Now his left ankle and foot were tilting left and right easily on the floor, almost like the right one.

"Keep turning and look at your left ankle now," I said.

"Hey, it's moving," he said. "But how come . . . Wait a minute. You're not going to tell me that whatever happened in my back made that ankle start moving, are you?"

"Well, if that wasn't it, wasn't it a funny coincidence that the ankle started to move just when you felt that motion in your back?"

"Yeah, well, I guess the important thing is that it's moving now. It feels funny, too, almost like it's bigger somehow," Bif said.

"Walk around a little and feel how the pressure moves

along the bottoms of your feet now," I suggested.

Bif began to walk back and forth. "The left foot has changed," he said. "Before, the pressure moved right up the center of the foot, and now it feels like it moves up the outside of the foot, almost like the right one." He walked some more, concentrating intensely on his feet. "On the right side the pressure goes right up through the little toe, but on the left side it goes up just between the little toe and the next one. It's a pretty small difference; I can hardly feel it."

Bif started to put on his shoes. "I want to go run and try it out," he said excitedly.

"Keep it down to 2 or 3 miles," I urged.

Twenty minutes later, Bif was back. "What happened?" I asked.

"My left knee still hurts," he said, "but it's not the same. I don't feel that pressure, and it's not stiff like it was before. What do you think?"

"I think that what you ought to do is not run for about three days, and then do some walking and light running for another three days, and then start building your mileage back up. Whatever it was that was hurting in your knee probably needs a few days to heal. How does that sound?"

Bif said that sounded good to him and that he would give me a call. Then he took off to go to a wedding.

The next week when I tried to get Bif on the phone, I found that he had gone out of town on business and I didn't hear from him for almost a month.

Finally, I got a call. "Twenty miles, and no pain," he said.

10

The Drive Point

In the foregoing chapters we have explored at length the parts of the body that have to move before we can run well. We've also explored some of the connections between these different parts. Now we're going to take all of this knowledge and put it together.

In this lesson you'll discover that the shoulders and the arms are the "drive point" for efficient running motion in the hips and legs. Because of the way the human body is structured, with its two-legged stance and so much of its weight held high up off the ground, the motion of the legs and hips must be counterbalanced by the motion of the arms and shoulders in order to generate power for running.

The connections that cause the motions of the upper body to balance the motions of the lower body are built into the nervous system. And interestingly enough, they work both ways, from the hips to the shoulders *and* from the shoulders to the hips.

We are going to activate this connection in the shoulder-to-hip direction, and you will learn to feel how the motion of the shoulders and arms can "drive" the feet. When this connection is well established, you'll feel that your legs have suddenly become stronger and that they move in a much more effective way than they ever have before. To begin, start to walk and pay particular attention to the right side of your body as your right foot moves forward to take a step. By now you should be able to feel clearly that as your right foot moves forward, the right hip also moves forward, and the right shoulder moves backward.

Briefly review the movement of the hips and shoulders that we have been working with since Chapter 1.

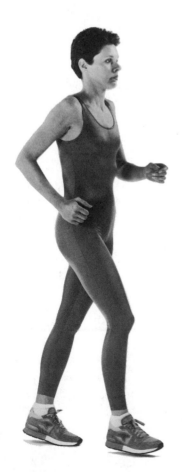

Photo 10-1: *Walk along with your elbows bent and your forearms almost horizontal, in the position that you use to run.*

To do this, first exaggerate the motion of the hips and shoulders for about 20 steps and then lock the hips and shoulders together and walk another 20 steps. Then exaggerate the hip and shoulder motion once more for another 20 steps, and finally just walk along in your usual way.

Continue to walk easily like this and bend your elbows so that your forearms are almost horizontal, in the position that you use to run. (Photo 10-1) As your right foot moves forward to take a step, while the foot is in the air, quickly snap your right elbow backward and let the right shoulder follow the elbow. (Photo 10-2) When the

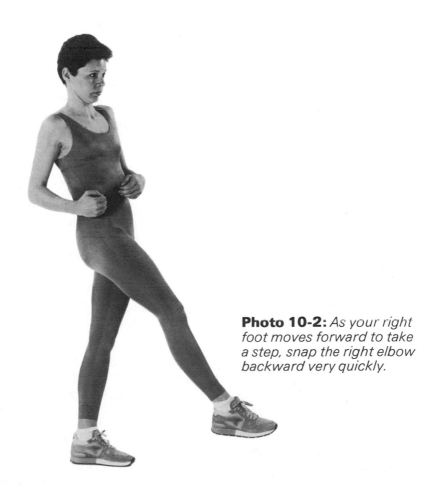

Photo 10-2: *As your right foot moves forward to take a step, snap the right elbow backward very quickly.*

left foot moves forward to take a step, let the arms and shoulders move in their usual way, then snap the right elbow backward again as the right foot moves forward to take a step, and so on. Be sure to let the left shoulder and arm move forward as the right shoulder snaps backward.

Continue to walk like this and make the motion of the right elbow and shoulder a quick, light, easy motion. As you snap the elbow back, notice what happens to the right leg and foot. Experiment with the timing of this snapping motion. Try snapping the right elbow backward just as the right foot leaves the ground; do this about 20 times. Then try snapping the elbow back just as the right foot is passing the left leg; do this 20 times also. Finally, snap the elbow back when the right foot is well ahead of the left leg and almost on the ground.

As you experiment with the timing of this movement, you will feel a connection between the snapping motion of the elbow and shoulder and a motion of the right hip, leg, and foot. As the elbow snaps back, the right foot will jump forward in a quick, kicking motion.

When you first feel this connection, the motion of the right foot will probably be small and tenuous, so you will have to pay careful attention to yourself and make light, easy motions to be able to recognize this movement of the foot. Nevertheless, when it comes, the feeling is unmistakable. The right foot will seem to jump forward almost by itself as the right elbow snaps back.

As this connection becomes clearer, you can increase the power of the arm and shoulder motion and notice how this increases the power of the leg and foot motion. Don't let yourself strain to do the motion, however. Keep your movements light and easy and make sure that you breathe easily as you move. Spend as much time as you want working with this, and then just walk along in your usual manner, directing your attention now to the left and right sides of your body. Do the two sides feel different?

Here is a second way to work with this connection between the upper and lower parts of the body. Stop walking and stand still in your usual standing posture. Leaving your left foot where it is on the floor, move your

right foot backward about 2 feet and to the right about
1 foot. Bend your left knee and straighten your right knee.
Make sure that you are facing straight forward, in the
direction that your left foot is pointing. Bend your elbows
so that your forearms are almost horizontal. (Photo 10-3)

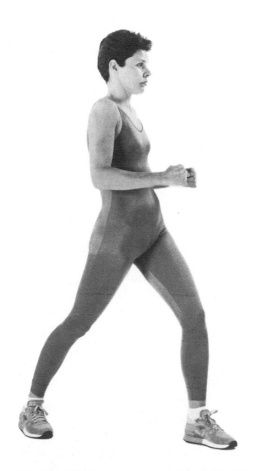

Photo 10-3: *Move your right foot backward about 2 feet
and to the right about 1 foot. Bend your left knee, straighten
your right knee, and bend your elbow so that your forearms
are horizontal.*

From this position, shift your weight forward and back a little, until you feel that about half your weight is on each foot.

Leaving your left foot where it is on the floor, bring your right foot forward and up. As the right foot passes the left leg, snap your right elbow and shoulder backward and let the right foot move forward in a kicking motion. (Photo 10-4) After the kick, reverse the sequence of motions and replace the right foot on the floor behind you. Don't let the right foot touch the floor in front after the kick.

Continue to work with this movement and notice how the motion of the arms and shoulders causes the right

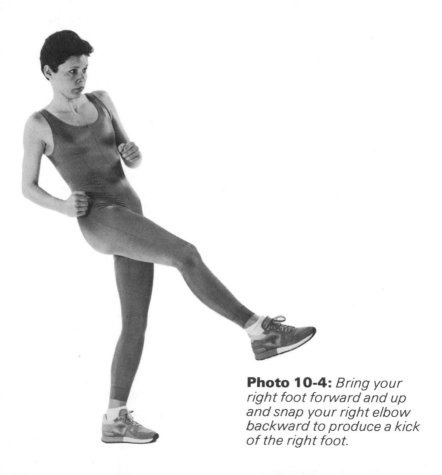

Photo 10-4: *Bring your right foot forward and up and snap your right elbow backward to produce a kick of the right foot.*

foot to snap out to make a kicking motion. As this connection becomes clearer to you, you'll find that the right foot kicks powerfully and that the right knee straightens out and locks at the end of the kick in front. To help you define this kicking motion, have a friend hold a piece of cardboard out in front at a comfortable level as a target for your kick. (Photo 10-5) As your kick improves, have your friend raise the height of the cardboard.

As you experiment with this motion, pay attention to what is going on in the rest of your body. Make sure that your breathing is easy and that you allow your shoulders and hips to move easily as you make the kick.

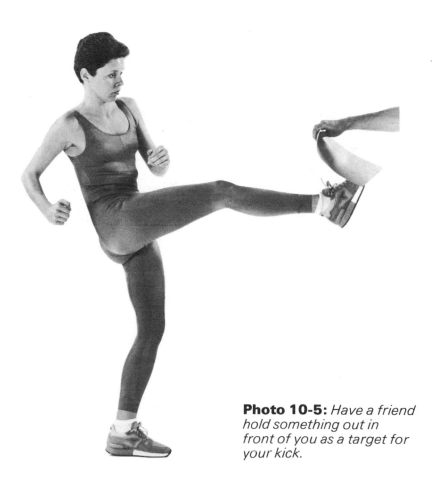

Photo 10-5: *Have a friend hold something out in front of you as a target for your kick.*

Try making the kicking motion a few times with the right knee straight, and then try it a few more times and bend the knee as much as you can as you bring the foot up to make the kick. Notice how these two variations affect the kick.

When you have spent some time experimenting with this kicking motion and have a good feeling for it, try reversing the motion of the shoulders. As you make the kick with the right foot, pull the *left* elbow and shoulder back and throw your right shoulder into the kick. (Photo 10-6) Make sure that you have plenty of room and a soft place to fall on, since you might fall when you try this.

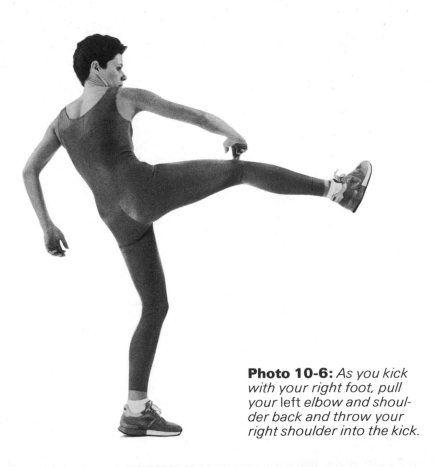

Photo 10-6: *As you kick with your right foot, pull your* left *elbow and shoulder back and throw your right shoulder into the kick.*

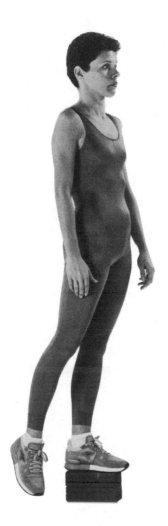

Photo 10-7: *Stand with your left foot on a couple of bricks or a thick book so that your right foot hangs down in the air.*

Throwing the right shoulder into the kick like this destroys the body's balance and actually ruins the whole motion. Rotating the shoulders in the opposite direction to the hips, however, allows the motion of the shoulders and arms to counterbalance the motion of the hips and legs, and makes the whole kicking movement easy, fluid, and elegant.

Go back and forth between the two motions of the shoulders a few times until the difference is clear to you.

Notice how experimenting with the "wrong" motion and getting a clear feel for just how it affects your kick actually improves the "right" motion.

After you have worked with the kick motion for a half-hour or so, go back and experiment with the first motion, when you were just walking along and moving the right shoulder and arm quickly back, and notice how much the motion has improved.

Here is yet another way to further refine and improve your sense of this upper-lower body connection. Stack up a couple of books or bricks on the floor or get a thick telephone book and set it on the floor to create a "step." Stand with your left foot on the step and your right foot hanging down in the air. The step should lift you high enough so that your right leg can hang down relaxed without the foot touching the floor. (Photo 10-7)

From this position, swing your right foot forward and back a little. Begin with a small motion, just moving the foot a couple of inches each way, and then gradually increase the motion. As you swing the foot, notice what you do with the rest of your body and pay particular attention to your shoulders and hips. Let your right hip move easily along with the foot, and let your right shoulder and arm move in the opposite direction to counterbalance the motion of the leg and hip. (Photos 10-8, 10-9)

This somewhat precarious position of standing on one foot allows you to feel exactly how the upper body must move to counterbalance the motion of the lower body. If the motion of any part is off just the least bit, you will lose your balance. This is a very precise way to gauge the efficiency of all your body movements. It actually allows you to fine-tune the motion.

As you swing the right leg forward, snap the right elbow and shoulder back. (Photo 10-10) At first, just increase the backward motion of the right arm slightly, and notice how the movement is transmitted through the hips to the right leg, and how the right foot snaps forward a little. Then speed up the backward motion of the right arm a little more, then a little more, and so on. If you find

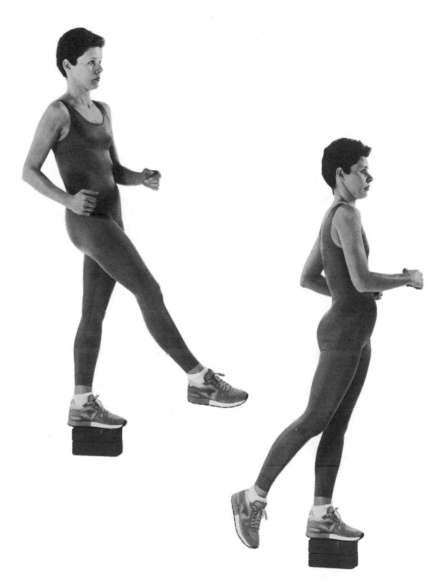

Photos 10-8, 10-9: *Swing your right leg forward and backward; counterbalance the motion of the lower body with the shoulders and arms.*

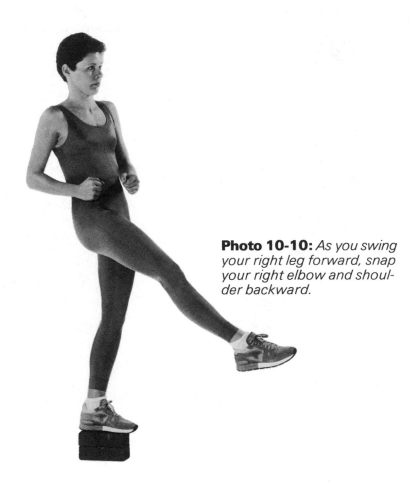

Photo 10-10: *As you swing your right leg forward, snap your right elbow and shoulder backward.*

that you start losing your balance or hold your breath as you do this, decrease the motion of the right arm a little and try to figure out which part of your body you are stiffening; this is actually what throws you off center and makes you start to fall. When you identify the stiff part, you will find that your balance improves, and that you can kick more powerfully without falling over.

After you have worked with this movement for 15 or 20 minutes, just walk along again and snap the right shoulder and arm backward. Do you notice any further improvement in the motion?

After all this, walk along and snap the right shoulder and arm backward as the right foot moves forward to take a step; then snap the left shoulder and arm backward as the left foot moves forward to take a step. Continue to walk like this for 20 or 30 steps. How big a difference can you feel between the two sides?

Take a break for 5 or 10 minutes and then repeat the three exercises, this time on the left side. Notice how quickly you progress on this side after learning the motion on the other side.

In the final chapter we'll take the motion that we learned here and integrate it into your running. Give yourself two or three days before you do the exercises in this last chapter, to enable your body to absorb what it has learned in this lesson. In the meantime review some of the moves in this lesson so that you will be well prepared for the final lesson.

Donna: A Disability Can Be an Asset

In class, Donna lay on her right side, moving her hips and shoulders forward and back, together and separately, and drawing circles first in one direction and then the opposite. She had quickly picked up on the idea that the purpose of the motions was to increase her awareness of how she was moving and not to stretch or strengthen the muscles. With that understanding, she progressed rapidly.

I watched her as she moved her hips and shoulders. Each move was slow and deliberate. I could see that her breathing was easy and that she was not straining or forcing the movements.

Donna had a special reason for being in the class. About 14 years before, at age 12, she had been thrown from a horse and had landed hard on her back. She had suffered some pain for a few days, but an examination by a doctor disclosed no serious injury, and after a few days

of rest she seemed to be all right except for a little
stiffness in her lower back.

In the ensuing years, however, her left thigh began to
degenerate. By the time I saw her, the left thigh, especially
the part near the knee, was less than half the size of the
right thigh. She could walk fairly well as long as she didn't
go too fast, but her running was just no good at all.

When she had signed up for the class, she told me all
this, and also told me that some of her friends had told her
that she "walked funny." She did feel that there was
something peculiar about the way that she walked and
that it was somehow caused by her accident, though she
couldn't quite put her finger on exactly what it was.

In the very first class we explored the motion of the
hips and shoulders while walking. When I asked everyone
to exaggerate the relative motion of the hips and shoulders as they walked, Donna seemed to have a real
problem doing it. I could see that she was doing just
about everything *but* exaggerating the motion of the
hips and shoulders.

When I asked everyone to lock the hips and shoulders
together, however, it was a different story. After a few
minutes of exploring this motion, Donna suddenly came
to a complete stop and said, "That's the way I walk all the
time. Ever since I fell off that horse."

She became so absorbed in her discovery that she
hardly listened for the rest of the class. Toward the end I
asked everyone to sit down while I talked about some
principles, and I could see her slowly moving her hips and
shoulders around, with tiny, almost imperceptible motions,
and her face had that faraway look that people get when
they are paying attention to some internal sensation.

Now we were coming to the end of the course, and at
the beginning of this session I had asked everyone to walk
along, trying to snap the right shoulder back very fast,
with the elbow bent, while the right foot was in the air to
take a step. After a half-hour of working with this, most of
the students had begun to feel that snapping the shoulder
back like this made the right foot jerk forward in a motion
almost like a kick. Nonetheless, no one seemed to feel the

connection clearly, and the class as a whole seemed dissatisfied.

After a short rest I asked the students to lie down on the floor on their right sides, and we began to move the left hip and shoulder about in various ways, exploring the way that the motion of the shoulder affected the hip and vice versa. Finally we drew circles with the left hip and shoulder. We went clockwise, then counterclockwise, and then tried various combinations of movements of the hip and shoulder.

After an hour of this I asked everyone to stand up and try the kicking motion on the left side. I asked them to notice the difference in the motion caused by exploring the movement of the hip and shoulder on the left side. Donna moved her left foot back on the floor, well behind her right, and tried the kick, snapping her left shoulder and elbow backward as she moved her left foot forward.

The effect was spectacular. Her left foot shot up off the floor, well over her head, and her knee extended with a snapping sound. It looked like the kind of kick that a karate black belt would do. Several people standing around her hurriedly moved back a few steps. Nobody wanted to be in range of that awesome kick.

Donna could hardly believe it, especially since her left leg was her bad one. I had her repeat the kick a few times, asking everyone to watch. As her foot shot up, her hips and shoulders moved in perfect sync, with the motion of the shoulders exactly counterbalancing the motion of the hips and left leg. It was really something to see. The kick had tremendous speed and power, yet Donna did not appear to be making an effort to do it. Thus inspired, everyone else suddenly found that they could also do the kick; but even after quite a bit of practice, no one could do it as well as Donna, not even some of the more athletic men.

Sometimes, those with a disability actually seem to learn faster than "normal" people. Donna had very weak thigh muscles and was unable to do the kick by means of strength. She just didn't have it. So she was forced to use her whole body in the most efficient way; otherwise she wouldn't have been able to do the movement at all.

Donna had discovered—in a spectacular way—that the shoulders and arms are the drive point, as I call it, for the motion of the foot and leg. What this means in practice is that once the muscles of your body are fairly well organized, if you want to move your feet quickly to do a kick or run fast, you should direct the effort into the shoulders and arms. Then the legs and feet will move almost by themselves. Once you have truly learned the motion, of course, you don't have to think of any particular part; you just do it.

Donna doesn't "walk funny" anymore, and even better, her left thigh has finally stopped shrinking and actually appears to have grown a little. Her doctor doesn't know why her thigh has begun to grow, but, of course, he didn't know why it had shrunk, either.

I think it has a lot to do with her "funny walk." As everyone knows, when a muscle is not used, it tends to degenerate. The most well-known example of this is seen when a limb is removed from a cast. Having been immobilized for a few weeks or months, the muscles that were under the cast are almost always shrunken and weak. Usually some special exercises for the affected limb restore strength and functioning without much trouble.

My idea is that because of Donna's "funny walk," caused by the injury to her back, the muscles of the left thigh were not being used and so they had slowly begun to shrink. When her walk changed, her muscles started to work again and to grow.

11

Running_____ _with the_____ _____Whole Body

In the previous lesson you discovered that the shoulders and arms are the drive point for the running motion of the legs. You learned to feel that making a quick, snapping motion backward with the arm and shoulder on one side causes the foot on that side to move forward in a motion like a kick.

This connection between the upper body and lower body is the key to good running. If, for some reason, the upper and lower parts do not work together, the motions of the heavy lower body will throw us off balance. Then we have to make a lot of unnecessary movements to try to keep ourselves upright, movements that interfere with our running.

But when this connection is working properly, the whole body runs in a balanced, efficient manner. Now you are going to learn to use this connection—the drive point—while you run, and you'll discover that you are a much better runner than you had ever dreamed you could be.

Start walking along in your normal manner and let your attention move through your body. Notice how your feet move, your knees, and then your hips. Let your attention move slowly up along your spine, through your chest and neck, and on up to your head. Notice how your shoulders move, and your elbows and hands.

Continue to walk and exaggerate the relative motion of the hips and shoulders. Again scan your body, noting how all the parts move. Then lock your hips and shoulders together and continue to walk. Once again, scan your body. Finally, return to your usual walk.

As you walk, imagine that your feet are leading the motion and that the rest of the body follows the feet. As you take a step, throw each foot quickly out in front in an exaggerated motion and let the rest of the body do whatever it has to do to help the foot. (Photo 11-1) Walk 200 to 300 feet like this until you have a clear feeling for the motion; then speed up and run, but not too fast, still letting the feet lead the motion.

This leads to a peculiar, showy kind of run that is not very fast or effective. Some people run like this all the time, though, and don't realize what they are doing. Run 100 feet like this and then slow down and walk, still letting the feet lead the motion. Then speed up and run once again, making sure that you pay attention to your whole body as you move. Run 20 or 30 paces like this as fast as you can, letting the feet lead the motion, and then slow down and walk along in your usual way. Can you feel any difference in your walk now? Stop walking and rest for a minute or two.

Walk along again and this time imagine that your knees are leading the motion. As you take a step, throw each knee quickly out in front in an exaggerated motion and let the rest of the body do whatever it has to do to

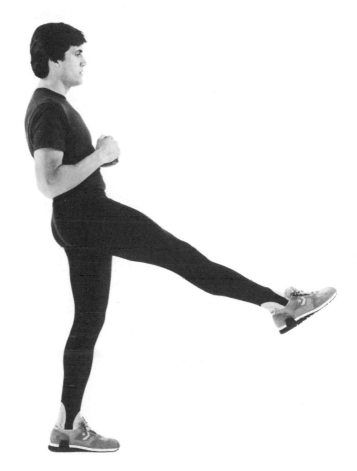

Photo 11-1: *Walk along and move your feet in an exaggerated movement forward so that they lead the walking motion.*

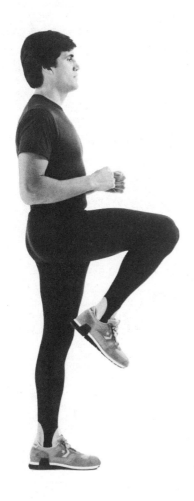

Photo 11-2: *Walk along and this time exaggerate the forward movement of your knees so that they lead the walking motion.*

help the knee. (Photo 11-2) Walk 200 to 300 feet like this until you have a clear feeling for the motion; then speed up and run, still letting the knees lead the motion.

Notice how this leads to a kind of running that is very different from the previous movement. This kind of running is relatively slow, but it's useful for running through obstacles, where not tripping is more important than speed. Run for 100 feet like this and then slow down and walk, still letting the knees lead the motion. Then speed up and run once again, making sure that you pay attention to your whole body as you move. Run for about

20 or 30 paces as fast as you can, letting your knees lead the motion, and then slow down and walk in your usual way. Can you feel any differences in your walk? Stop walking and rest for a minute or two.

Again begin to walk along, and this time imagine that your hips lead the motion. As you take a step, throw each hip quickly out in front in an exaggerated motion and let the rest of the body do whatever it has to do to help the hip move. (Photo 11-3) Walk 200 to 300 feet like this until you have a clear feeling for the motion, and then speed up and run, still letting the hips lead the motion.

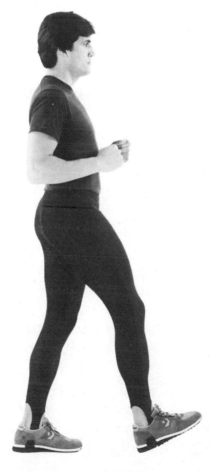

Photo 11-3: *Walk along, this time exaggerating the forward movement of your hips so that they lead the walking motion.*

Notice how this leads to a third kind of running, very different from the previous two. Many women and some men who do not run well run like this. It is a pretty ineffective way of running, on the whole, but it's worth trying just as a learning experience, to find out how it feels. Remember in Lesson 10, when you practiced the "wrong way" of kicking and improved the "right way" in the process? Can you learn something about the right way of running from this? Run for about 100 feet like this and then slow down and walk. Make sure that the hips

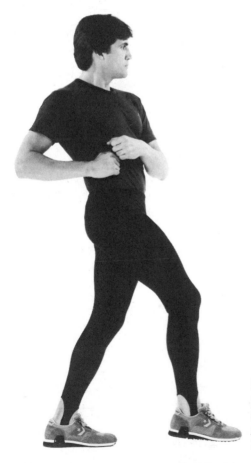

Photo 11-4: *This time as you walk, move the arms and shoulders in an exaggerated movement so that they lead the walking motion.*

continue to lead the motion. Walk for a while, then speed up and run again. Run for about 20 or 30 paces as fast as you can, again letting the hips lead the motion, and then slow down and walk again. How does your walk feel now? Stop walking and rest for a few minutes.

Start walking again and now imagine that your shoulders and arms lead the motion. As you take a step, throw each shoulder and arm back in a quick, snappy, exaggerated motion, and let the rest of the body do whatever it has to do to allow the shoulders and arms to lead. (Photo 11-4) Walk 200 to 300 feet like this until you have a good feeling for the motion; then speed up and run, but don't go too fast.

Notice what kind of running this leads to. You will feel that this gives the smooth, powerful run of a natural athlete. Run for about 200 or 300 feet like this and then slow down and walk. Make sure that your shoulders and arms are still leading the motion.

Once again speed up, shoulders and arms leading the motion, until you are running at a slow jogging speed. Jog about 200 feet and then very quickly accelerate the motion of your shoulders and arms until they are moving as fast as you can move them.

Run for 20 or 30 paces like this, then slow down and walk. After a short walk, repeat the previous sequence, speeding up to a slow jogging speed, running about 200 feet, and then accelerating the motion of the shoulders and arms.

Notice what happens when you accelerate the shoulders and arms like this. You will probably feel that you have been suddenly shot out of a cannon. The incredible sensations of acceleration and speed produced by running like this, especially the first time you do it, are almost indescribable. Many people actually feel as if they are suddenly going *too* fast and have to hold themselves back.

After you have experienced these sensations while running, try to get them beginning from a standing start. Notice how much faster you can accelerate to your top speed by using the shoulders and arms to lead the motion.

Rich: Nothing to It

I stood in the park with Rich. It had been just over nine months since we had first come to this park, the day he had almost given himself a stroke by running the grand distance of 200 feet. That nine months had been one of my most frustrating and difficult teaching experiences. Rich had decided that he was going to learn to run, come hell or high water, but his body didn't seem to be interested in his decision.

Every time I would come up with a new technique to improve Rich's running, he would find a dozen different ways to do it incorrectly. If his legs started to move a little better, he would freeze up his shoulders. If I loosened his shoulders, he would find a way to make his breathing difficult. When he finally started to breathe normally again, he had lost the improvement in his legs.

Once I asked him why he was suddenly so determined, at 38 years of age, to learn to run when he had never put much time or energy into it before.

"But I did put a lot of time and energy into it," Rich protested. "I just never knew what to do. All the people I asked about it said I should just try harder, or practice more, or run with some better runners, or breathe deeper, or . . . you know what I mean. I had pretty much given up on running until I found you.

"Then on that first day over here, when you got me to feel how my right hip moved forward when my right foot moved forward, it was like some kind of window opened up inside me. All of a sudden I knew, somehow, that that was what had been missing.

"And that's what has kept me going all these months. I want to find out what happens when I get all the parts to work together in the right way. It's like solving some kind of puzzle.

"And there's another thing, too," he continued. "All the other stuff I tried was like something imposed on me from the outside, and I didn't really like it. It was like I was doing it for other people, running *their* way. This way, the way that you teach, is exactly the opposite. It seems to come from the inside out. And somehow, that makes all the difference."

Rich had taken my running class three times. The first time he took it, he told me later, I might as well have been speaking Greek. The idea of paying attention to his body and learning from the "inside out," as he put it—in fact, my whole approach to learning to run—were so foreign to his way of thinking that it just didn't make any sense to him at all.

The second time he took the class, he began to get an idea of what I was talking about. In addition, watching some of the other people learn provided some real inspiration for him.

The third time, everything began to click. Not only could he feel the individual parts of his body and how they moved while he walked and ran, but he was actually beginning to feel some of the connections that I talked about. Moving the shoulders in a certain way really did cause the foot to make a motion like a kick, and the hip joint really did have to be free for the ankle and foot to work properly.

Gradually, over the months, Rich began to loosen up. He felt good enough now to do a little easy jogging two or three evenings a week, and, incredibly, he told me, his back and legs didn't hurt the next morning.

And so today I had come with Rich once more to the park. As we walked along I had him review the motions of his hips and shoulders. I could see that his motions were easy and fluid now, and that he had a good feeling for all the movements of the different parts of his body. I knew this because he could move his hips and shoulders together or separately and go back and forth between the two motions with ease. I had a feeling that Rich was ready.

I began to talk Rich through the last lesson, starting with exaggerating the movements of his feet while walking. After that we worked with the knees and then the hips. In each case, I had him exaggerate the motions while walking, then speed up and run, then walk again, then run again, and so on. I went through each movement four or five times. I didn't want to take any chances with Rich.

Finally we worked our way up to the shoulders. I had Rich run slowly, leading with the shoulders, and then very gradually speed up just a little, while I watched for signs of stiffness or straining. When I didn't see any, I had him speed up just a little more. Still he seemed to be running smoothly and easily. I judged that the time was right.

I walked along with Rich and told him what I wanted him to do. "Run along like you have been doing, at a medium pace, for 20 or 30 steps. Make sure that you let your shoulders lead the motion. Then speed up the motion of your arms and shoulders, very quickly, until they are moving as fast as they can."

Rich took off and I watched with some trepidation. This was the point where he had always failed before. When he sensed that he was going to make an effort, he would stiffen up his whole body, and his running motion would fall apart.

At a certain point I saw Rich speed up his arms and shoulders, and for a second I thought that he had succumbed to his old habits and let himself get stiff again. He seemed to stumble and almost fall, but then he kept going, and suddenly his whole running motion changed. He stood up straight and began to run with very quick, short, high steps, almost like a veteran running back dodging opposing tacklers.

Rich ran around in a wide arc and came back to where I was standing, still using that sort of strange-looking running motion. I could see that there had been a big change for the better in Rich's running, but I was baffled by his high steps. None of my students had ever done that before.

"What happened?" I asked.

Rich had a strange, intense look on his face. His elbows were still bent and his hands were clenched into fists as if he were still running. "When I started to move my shoulders like you said, I felt myself begin to stiffen up," he said. "But all of a sudden I could feel exactly what I was doing to make myself stiff, and I just realized that I could let go of it, and I did. It threw me off, and I almost fell down.

"And then, I felt my legs take off, and it was *scary!* I felt like I was going to go so fast that I wouldn't be able to handle it. So I kind of held back my legs."

"Go try it again," I said, "and see if you can let your feet move forward without picking them up so high."

Rich took off, still using that strange, high-stepping motion. He ran about 200 feet and then circled around a tree and started back toward me. He made a tight turn and leaned so far into it that it looked as if he were going to fall over sideways.

Rich came out of the turn like a freight train that had lost its brakes on a steep grade. The high-stepping motion was gone and he was running as if the devil himself were hot on his heels. He was heading straight toward me, and I suddenly had a strong desire to jump out of his way. I had the feeling that a brick wall wouldn't slow Rich down much just then.

I quickly moved sideways a few steps, just as Rich tore past me. I could hear him laughing under his breath. He ran another 50 feet, slowed down to a walk, and came back to where I was standing. He was still chuckling.

"What's so funny?" I asked.

"It was so damned *easy*, after all these years of trying," he said. "In fact, it would be hard *not* to run fast. I'd have to hold myself back. In fact, that's just what I've been doing all these years. Holding myself back, I mean. But once you can feel it, all you have to do is let go."

I wanted to make sure that Rich had it all down pat, so I asked him, "If you had to describe what you felt, how would you do it?"

Rich hesitated briefly before answering. "It's the shoulders and arms that make the whole thing go," he said. "And now I can feel what all that work that we did in class was for. When I went around that tree, I realized that I wasn't going to fall and I let the motion of the upper body go down through my hips to my feet. And then I just took off. Nothing to it."

About the Feldenkrais Method

The Feldenkrais Method was developed by Moshe Feldenkrais, D.Sc., during the middle part of this century. After a serious injury to one knee during a soccer match in France in 1926, at the age of 22, Feldenkrais began a search for a way to rehabilitate his defective knee. He studied physics and electrical engineering at the Sorbonne, where he earned a doctor of science degree. When the Germans invaded France in 1940, Feldenkrais went to England, where he helped to develop what we now call sonar.

While he was in France, Feldenkrais was introduced to Jigoro Kano, the founder of Judo; his meeting with Kano inspired him to earn a black belt and form Le Judo Club de France. During all this time, he continued his search for a way to improve the use of his knee. It finally led him to investigate the importance of movement learning in human beings. Drawing on his theoretical experience in physics and engineering and his practical experience in judo, he began to experiment on himself. He gradually discovered ways that allowed him to improve the use of his knee.

As his investigations continued, he found that moving and thinking were closely linked. As a result, he started to study the emotional and mental aspects of human functioning and how they related to posture and movement. The outcome of those investigations was published in his theoretical book, *Body and Mature Behavior,* in 1949.

His ideas about human functioning and how to improve it were considered radical at that time, however, and were not well received. So Feldenkrais returned to Israel, where he had lived before moving to France, and continued to work as an engineer. Fortunately, he also continued to develop his method of movement education, and gradually word began to leak out of Israel that an extraordinary man was working physical wonders for people with a method of his own devising.

Feldenkrais found that he could help other people to function better in the same way that he had helped himself. He gradually began to devote more and more of his time to his work in movement education. As his fame spread, many people interested in improving their own ways of moving sought him out. Those injured by stroke, accident, or disease found that they could learn to sit, stand, walk, and talk again after working with Feldenkrais's method. Athletes, dancers, and musicians discovered that the method could actually make them perform better with less pain and effort.

The list of well-known people who have worked with Feldenkrais is impressive. It includes violinist Yehudi Menuhin, classical guitarist Narcisco Yepes, conductor Igor Markevitch, and basketball player Julius Erving, better known as "Dr. J" to his fans. In addition, Feldenkrais taught at the International Center of Theatre Research in Paris, France, the Brooklyn Academy of Music, the drama school at New York University, and many other institutions of learning throughout the world.

The method developed by Feldenkrais consists of two parts, which are known as Awareness Through Movement and Functional Integration. Awareness Through Movement is taught in groups. In a class, the students sit or lie on the floor and the teacher gives verbal directions for exercises. Each lesson gives the student an opportunity to gently and slowly explore some aspect of his physical functioning. This exploration results in improved awareness, greater flexibility, increased range of movement, better posture, and better breathing. Feldenkrais's best-known book, *Awareness Through Movement,* published in 1972, explains this part of his method in detail and gives 12 lessons so that the reader can experience the method firsthand.

Functional Integration is taught individually. In a session, the student lies on a padded table; the teacher then uses his or her hands to guide the student into new and better patterns of movement. Although the method is not therapy, many people who work with it find relief from a variety of aches and pains.

Before his death in 1984, Feldenkrais conducted three programs to train others to do his work. Current training programs are conducted by his senior students.

As of this writing there are about 2,000 authorized Feldenkrais teachers in the world, with another 1,000 students in training programs. The Feldenkrais Guild, an organization of the teachers of this method, was established by Feldenkrais himself in 1977. The Guild maintains a directory of those who have completed an authorized Professional Training Program and are qualified to do the work. For more information about the Guild, please write to The Feldenkrais Guild, P.O. Box 489, Albany, OR 97321, or call (800) 775-2118.

About the Author

Jack Heggie earned a degree in physics and worked as a digital computer design engineer, programmer, and field engineer for ten years before becoming a Feldenkrais Practitioner. He studied with Dr. Feldenkrais in Israel and the US, and has trained with Ruthy Alon, Mia Segal, and Shlomo Efrat, all senior Feldenkrais trainers. Heggie has written about the Feldenkrais approach of learning through awareness for *Skiing, NorthWest Skier, Boston SportScape, Snow Country, The Instrumentalist, Direction,* and *Somatics* magazines. He maintains a private practice in Boulder, Colorado and Dallas, Texas. Mr. Heggie is available to teach running and skiing workshops. He may be contacted at the Boulder Center for the Feldenkrais Method, 2888 Bluff Street, Suite 134, Boulder, CO 80301.

Bibliography

Books by Moshe Feldenkrais, DSc.

Practical Unarmed Combat. London: Frederick Warne, 1941

Judo: The Art of Defense and Attack. London: Frederick Warne, 1944.

Body and Mature Behavior: A Study of Anxiety, Sex, Gravitation, and Learning. NY: International Universities Press, 1949.

Higher Judo (Groundwork). London: Frederick Warne, 1952.

Awareness Through Movement: Health Exercises for Personal Growth. NY/London: Harper & Row, 1972.

The Case of Nora: Body Awareness As Healing Therapy. Berkeley, CA: Somatic Resources/Frog, Ltd., 1993.

The Elusive Obvious. Cupertino, CA: Meta Publications, 1981.

The Master Moves. Cupertino, CA: Meta Publications, 1984.

The Potent Self: A Guide to Spontaneity. NY: Harper & Row, 1985.

Books By Other Authors

Mindful Spontaneity, Ruthy Alon. Berkeley, CA: North Atlantic Books, 1993.

Relaxercise, David and Kaethe Zemach-Bersin, and Mark Reese. NY: Harper & Row, 1990.

The Body of Life, Thomas Hanna. NY: Knopf, 1980.

Somatics, Thomas Hanna. Reading, MA: Addison-Wesley, 1988.

The Use of the Eyes in Movement, Jack Heggie. Berkeley,
    CA: Feldenkrais Resources, 1985.

Skiing with the Whole Body, Jack Heggie. Berkeley, CA:
    North Atlantic Books, 1993.

The Feldenkrais Method: Teaching by Handling, Yochanan
    Rywerant. NY: Giniger/Harper & Row, 1983.